This is a story of a mom who believed in the ability of her son and in the ability of a community to embrace him. Led by her strong spiritual faith, she gently guided a community into a state of acceptance and then marveled at the ease with which they responded.

One tiny chromosome would not defeat her and her son.

Sue Maner
Executive Vice President
Special Olympics South Carolina

Martha, I have just completed "Down Strong" on my way back from New Jersey. I have also completed approximately one and a half boxes of tissues...(thank you very much)

It is amazing how much one can learn and one can teach even after 47 years on this planet.

Your book was eye-opening...enlightening...entertaining...comical...and most of all...heartfelt. I now have a beautiful new outlook on myself..my family..my friends...and all who I have yet to meet in life.

Trampus's story is a journey through a beautiful life...all while learning at the same time. You have shown that love...faith..courage..and resolve can only have one understand what is possible in life...what can be imagined...and most of all what can be accomplished... you have gifted the limitless potential in all of us.. and for that...I thank you.

Leo Rosten once said..."THE PURPOSE OF LIFE IS TO MATTER...TO COUNT...TO STAND FOR SOMETHING...TO HAVE IT MAKE SOME SENSE THAT YOU'VE LIVED AT ALL" Your story has demonstrated this in the clearest and brightest of colors.

I am proud to be your friend...I am proud to have had the opportunity to meet "the inner man". In more ways than one.

God bless you for blessing us...Joe Spiotta

Joe Spiotta, Owner
Bricco Bracco Italian Restaurant
Mount Pleasant, South Carolina

CHARLESTON SOUTHERN UNIVERSITY

VICE PRESIDENT FOR STUDENT AFFAIRS AND ATHLETICS

WOW! What a Story! WOW! What a family!! If you're looking for a real story about REAL faith and family here it is.

Just like his namesake, Billy Sunday, Trampus is an "evangelist" for hope and perseverance. His life "shouts" unconditional love and joy. I know, because I'm one of his "parishioners." One cannot be around Trampus, Martha, Vince and Tripp very long without being inspired and energized by their faith and genuine love for God, each other, and their "neighbor."

Rick Brewer, PhD, MBA

DOWN STRONG

MARTHA STEWART HOOVER

DOWN STRONG

The Amazing Life of
William Sunday Trampus Hoover

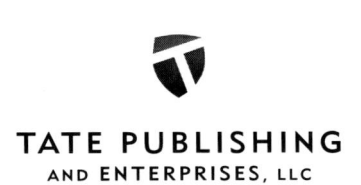

TATE PUBLISHING
AND ENTERPRISES, LLC

Down Strong
Copyright © 2014 by Martha Stewart Hoover. All rights reserved.

No part of this publication may be reproduced, stored in a retrieval system or transmitted in any way by any means, electronic, mechanical, photocopy, recording or otherwise without the prior permission of the author except as provided by USA copyright law.

The opinions expressed by the author are not necessarily those of Tate Publishing, LLC.

Published by Tate Publishing & Enterprises, LLC
127 E. Trade Center Terrace | Mustang, Oklahoma 73064 USA
1.888.361.9473 | www.tatepublishing.com

Tate Publishing is committed to excellence in the publishing industry. The company reflects the philosophy established by the founders, based on Psalm 68:11,
"The Lord gave the word and great was the company of those who published it."

Book design copyright © 2014 by Tate Publishing, LLC. All rights reserved.
Cover design by Jim Villaflores
Interior design by Gram Telen

Published in the United States of America

ISBN: 978-1-63185-341-8
1. Family & Relationships / Children With Special Needs
2. Family & Relationships / Parenting / General
14.04.30

This is the story of a mother taking her child's diagnosis with Down syndrome, and allowing her family, community, and faith to work it for good.

CONTENTS

Foreword 13

Preface 15

Introduction 17

Conception 19

First Six Weeks 27

Six Months 35

Toddler 39

Preschool 45

Preschool/Kindergarten 53

Elementary School 61

Middle School 111

High School 131

College 151

Life After School 167

FOREWORD

Trampus was the first of our special needs children at Whiteside's Elementary School. In many ways, he was our pioneer. I felt I learned so much from him and his family on how to support, not only special needs children, but all children and their individual differences and needs.

The Hoover family helped me to see that the best way to help any child is through a partnership of all of his or her stakeholders, family members, teachers, other students, community members and administrators. The Hoover family never demanded anything, but always asked how we as school personnel along with them could best help Trampus. This was the approach that we used throughout Trampus' career at Whiteside's and is what we strived to do with every child who came to the school after him.

I quickly learned that those parents who came to us demanding various services rather than trying to build partnerships were the ones whose children were less successful. Trampus and his family had a lasting impact on the teachers and staff at Whiteside's Elementary School because his successes gave us the confidence to believe that we could take on other special needs children and help them too.

In the coming years our doors were filled with many special needs children who were very successful and I can't help but believe that many of the lessons we learned with Trampus helped us to be successful with other children too.

Blessings,

Dave Schlacter
Former Principal
Whitesides Elementary School

PREFACE

What you are about to read is the story of a young man, William Sunday Trampus Hoover, who has Down syndrome. We call him Trampus. It is the story of a person taking what he has been given, and using it as an asset. This story is about what family really means, and you will find within these pages, some of the inspiring experiences of individuals whose lives have been touched through their moments with Trampus. You see, we have found that the life of one with Down syndrome does not have to be wrought with disqualifications, restrictions or even disadvantages. ALL that Trampus is has been a precious gift our entire family treasures. My daughter called me one day and asked if I had ever googled my name... I had not. She said, "Well google your name and then google Trampus Hoover. Try it and you will see what I mean when I say "taking what he has been given and using it as an asset".

The documentation began in journal form. As I chronicled our days and experiences with Trampus, friends began to hear about it and encouraged me to share it. The thought was there, but I never got around to actually pursuing it. My oldest granddaughter, who has entered the professional world, and will one day start a family of her own, requested a copy. After reading it, she told me that it gave her a new prospective about how children, all children, should be reared. She felt very strongly that it should be made available to others.

Thank you Emily for your encouragement and love in this project. Thank you, Martha Lucas, for your endless hours of editing and constant support. And thank all of you who have been a vital part of this journey.

I hope your life will be enriched by this book and more importantly, that you are encouraged to see that our greatest gifts of wisdom, understanding, perseverance and especially love come to us in the most amazing and sometimes unlikely ways when we are willing to open our eyes and our hearts.

I love you William Sunday Trampus Hoover, and thank God for every thought of you!! Martha Stewart Hoover.

INTRODUCTION

Our much desired baby became a part of our family on our chosen date of May 1, 1987. This date is celebrated for bringing forth new life…May day. But it would soon become the international sign for help…Mayday, Mayday. A dear friend, Carol Barrett, who shared in the excitement and anticipation of this new life, went with me into surgery. I remember hearing "he's very small" and feeling the first twinge of emotion. Is that significant? So what! I'm not big. Are you trying to tell me something? The doctor commented that he looked good and that they would bring him to me when I got out of recovery and back to my room. I really don't remember that period of time, but I do remember the nurse telling me that my husband was rocking the baby. When the pediatrician came into my room later that evening, I could see concern on his face. As he walked over to my side, I heard the words, "Martha, I think the baby may have the extra chromosome." It was like a knife cutting into my heart. I couldn't seem to catch my breath. I kept thinking this is a cruel joke, right? With so much discussion about my age and the possibility of having a baby with Down syndrome, had it now become a reality? It had to be a joke. Why the very thing people had warned us about? Why the very thing I seemed to be most fearful about? Why not spinal bifida, cerebral palsy? Why Down syndrome? My battle had begun—"my sought after gift" from God appeared to be damaged.

Before I continue with our journey, allow me to explain a little about myself along with some of the facts that led up to the desire for this baby. Let me introduce you to some of the people that have helped in this journey that began in fear and confusion, but has been transformed into a beautiful experience of hope, joy, and success.

CONCEPTION

For many years, my happiness and contentment was based on the influence of what others determined as fulfilling (i.e., the importance of furthering my education, where I lived, the car I drove, and who I chose as friends). Rather than searching my own heart, I tried to exist from outside input. Thankfully, I am married to a strong man who is caring and more committed to his family than myself. He was able to stand by me as I tried to look within for answers.

While my childhood experience included the church, there was no understanding of a personal day-to-day relationship with the One who created me. I knew about the faith that I had been given; however, that faith was weak just like an unused muscle. Exercising that faith can be as uncomfortable as having to exercise the muscles. Without it, they will atrophy. Once my eyes were opened to the fact that the loving and forgiving God who made me desired this faith to grow, I began to go to His Word for instruction. With this new life awakened within me, and His Words that began to provide guidance, I found myself discovering other women experiencing the same. We began to meet together and study the Scriptures. Out of this Scripture study, came a friendship I not only treasure, but still need today. She is my dear friend and prayer partner Judy Pezanowski. She has been by my side not only as supporter, encourager, and comforter, but most importantly as my intercessor (one who prays on behalf of another).

All of us were searching, but one area of concern that seemed universal was the raising of our children. In this one aspect of my life, I had enjoyed and experienced both worldly and personal "success." I was able to encourage my fellow Bible study students to experience what I had found. According to God's Word, children were a gift, their well-being would be great, and love never failed. Some were struggling with rebellious teenagers who were shaving their heads, rebelling at home, and challenging any type of authority. I would try to stress the need to love just as we would want to be loved. I would explain to them to just accept these children as gifts from God and then allow Him to guide the way.

This seemed so obvious to me. After all, I had a fourteen-year-old, blonde, blue-eyed daughter who responded on demand. She was an excellent student and had the love and talent for sports that her father desired. My six-year-old son was brown-haired, brown-eyed, and handsome like his daddy. He loved to please all those around him, and was now ready "to leave me" and begin school on a full-time basis. Becoming a full-time mom was quickly becoming a part-time job. Evaluating the now and anticipating the future caused me to conclude that my dwindling roll as a full-time, homebound mother was undesirable to me, and could not provide the success I had enjoyed up to this point.

I had been feeling this desire to have a baby for a long time but just mentioned it now and then. Most people's response was, "Why would you want to be tied down again now that your children will be in school all day?" My husband's initial reaction was negative as well. Finally, I asked God to either take the desire for a baby away, or put the desire in my husband also. I knew that becoming a mother again would require help from God since I had a tubal ligation after my last child and it was doubtful it could be reversed. If it could be reversed, becoming pregnant was not a guarantee. I realized my husband's change of heart when he mentioned that there was a gynecologist in our town who specialized in fertilization problems. Believing God was in this change of heart, I was sure my opportunity for continued success and contentment was not over.

We made an appointment and went through the exam. The doctor determined the operation could be performed successfully. My husband's first request was that we name our new baby after his uncle Billy. I have always wondered how he was so sure it would be a boy. Of course I agreed, and immediately contacted my mother-in-law to get the details of her brother's name. She told me he had been named after the evangelist Billy Sunday. So our new family member would be named William Sunday Hoover, or at least I thought it was. Before we officially signed off on this name, my husband informed me that we would be adding "Trampus." One of our friends, the Gladdens, had all girls and knew there would be no more children. Danny had always wanted to name a boy Trampus after one of the stars in the western series *The Virginian*. Danny put in the request and the decision was made; his name would be William Sunday Trampus Hoover.

After the surgery, my husband had to go to France on business so I went with him. We were on a dinner boat cruise when he pulled out a notepad from a hotel he always stayed when in New York, and jotted something down. He passed it over to me and my heart jumped as I read, "Going down the Seine with you and Billy Sunday. I love you." All I could think of was what a wonderful gift to give a child—a note from a father expressing his love for him before he was even conceived.

Just as I had expected, the surgery proved to be successful and my much-desired little one was on his way.

We had discussed as a family the realization that having a baby at forty years old left us vulnerable to a child with an extra chromosome. We all came to the same conclusion—it didn't matter. We wanted another family member! Fortunately, the other family members had sincerely searched their hearts (the inner man) and their minds (the soul) and had truthfully come into agreement within themselves that it didn't matter. Unfortunately, I realized after the fact, that I had not—but rather had left my inner man out of it and decided with my mind (soul) that since I had lost my first baby after only four days of life, it just wouldn't happen to me.

Because my other children were born via cesarean section, it was determined that this one should be as well. The date was set for May 1, 1987. Since I was sure Trampus was the miracle work of God in changing the heart of my husband for a baby, I was anxiously awaiting his arrival.

I guess because I believed this baby was truly the result of a miracle, hearing the heart-wrenching news of the possibility that our new baby may have Down syndrome seemed impossible. My husband quietly listened as the genetic specialist evaluated our son, Trampus: "he would likely stop developing by age eight," "we would have him for life." My first thought was, I can't handle this—I don't know how. I'm scared. I've never known anyone with DS or even been around anyone with DS. I imagined that this baby might not walk or be able to communicate with others. I was concerned over pictures I had seen, and sadly enough, I was already feeling embarrassed. I was totally overwhelmed.

As my heart was racing and the battle was raging between my mind and my inner man, I felt something coming up from deep within me. I was reflecting on my own words from the past while teaching the other mothers—just love him. This should have been much easier for me than it was for them since he hadn't shaved his head or cursed at me. I now needed to do what I had been encouraging others to do. The saddest thing at this point was I had allowed this news to steal my joy over the birth of this precious baby. The heaviness was felt not only by us, but the hospital staff as well. It was as if everyone was struggling—not sure what to say. I had already had three children, and I knew that everyone normally was excited about the new babies; everyone that came in would usually express their congratulations. This time, however, we didn't see the smiles of excitement, but faces that reflected pity and concern.

As the doctor stood by, I looked helplessly and fearfully at my husband to see his reaction. After all, Trampus was initially my heart's desire. He responded with such authority: "What is my son's physical condition? His heart? His respiration?" etc. The doctor stated that everything looked good. He couldn't see any real problems as far as his physical health was concerned. The most wonderful words a mother could hear came from my husband, "Then you have not told me anything that we can't take care of and I hope that you are right…in fact, I would hope that I could have all of my children at home with me for the rest of my life." Slowly but surely, I was beginning to be able to allow what was inside to control what was coming in through my mind. I began to remember Scriptures such as "I can do all things through Christ who strengthens me" (Philippians 4:13, NKJV), "no weapon formed against you shall prosper" (Isaiah 54:17, NKJV), and that "God is able to make all grace (help) abound unto you (2 Corinthians 9:8 NKJV). I knew at this point it was time for a serious exercise program with my faith to begin. It was time to practice walking by faith and not by sight.

The next step was to determine how to tell the children, our families, and friends. After all, some had questioned us to this possibility and wondered why we would pursue something that could end this way.

Our children were so excited about the baby and their eyes just sparkled every time they looked at him. We didn't say anything to them while we were in the hospital. I'm not sure I could have talked about it even if we had decided to tell them then.

Three days after Trampus was born, it suddenly occurred to me that I had not heard a word from a dear friend, Norma Kulseth, who had been with me all through this pregnancy. I had been in the delivery room when her baby, my godchild, was born, so where was she? It came to me quickly—her nephew had Down syndrome. We had talked very little about him, and I see now how even when we did, I was not really listening. It didn't affect me; it wasn't a concern of mine. Suddenly, I remembered something about battles her sister-in-law had with getting him in programs, etc. Now I wanted to hear. Where was this friend right now when I needed her? Later, when we were able to talk, I found out that the heaviness we were experiencing was extended out into the community as well. She was dealing with confusion and needed a little time to deal with her emotions. She said she found herself making excuses for delaying her visit to the hospital. I think her husband's statement "you need to get over there" is what really pressed her into coming. (It is amazing how the fear of the unknown can have such a paralyzing effect.) While Norma was aware of Trampus's birth, she felt as did others, we had "drawn the curtains." While I admit I had done that within, I had not intended to do the same to others around us.

By that afternoon, the door opened and she walked in with a large present. There was such understanding on her face and she didn't say anything. She just hugged me and told me to open the present. As I pulled the paper off of a beautifully framed picture, these words leapt into view, "God Danced the Day You were Born. You are loved, You are beautiful, You are a gift of God, His own possession. You are a gift to all mankind, His gift of love to them. You are His. William Sunday Hoover, May 1, 1987." She had ordered this long before his birth since the date and first choice for his name had already been decided. What an incredible confirmation to what I was hearing inside! The assurance of God's confirmation: you shouldn't go by the appearance of things on the outside and you shouldn't lean on your own understanding. Accept His promise that children are a gift from Him. She will never know or really understand what that gift meant then and continues to mean as we raise this precious gift from God.

FIRST SIX WEEKS

The first week we were home was probably the most difficult for me. The fear of the unknown was in my face all of the time. I would catch myself questioning God and my faith.

I decided it was time for me to deal with all the thoughts in my mind screaming "damaged." As I played out my conversation in my mind, I thought, *Okay, I would just ask God for his healing.* As the mental exercise progressed, I could hear from deep inside the question, *What needs to be healed?* My first request would be to heal his mind; allow him to be intellectually gifted like his brother and sister. But then the words from the Scripture echoed to me, "You have hidden these things from the wise and prudent and have revealed them to babes" (Matthew 11:25 NKJV). While I knew that this Scripture was not saying God doesn't bless us with intelligence, it reminded me that we don't need intellect to be all that He called us to be. I remembered that since He was not a respecter of persons, He gave each of us a spirit of power, of love, and of a "sound mind." Resolved! My second request began to manifest in my mind—how he looked. Once again the Scripture rose up, "Do not judge according to appearance but judge with righteous judgment" (John 7:24 NKJV). So much for his physical attributes.

Just to make sure I had covered everything, I pursued the extra chromosome and the possibility of getting rid of it. As far as I could understand, this syndrome was a chromosome problem. The next thought settled all of my fears and pleading for healing. Since when did something extra take away from what was already there? At this point, I knew in my heart that the gift that was little Trampus was not damaged, but rather he was given to me as a good and perfect gift to help complete what was lacking in me, and those involved in "my world."

My thoughts then moved on to Vince and his approach to this baby. Did he mean what he said when he told the doctor "as long as he had good health, we could take care of the rest?" I found myself wondering why had he been the one that was so strong and without fear. I was the one studying Scripture, leading Bible studies, and professing my faith so boldly. I finally determined that he had been living his beliefs and faith, while I was obviously just talking about mine.

I'll never forget one night Vince had gone out to run an errand. When he returned, I was stretched out on our bed with the baby beside me. He lay down next to me and somehow I knew that he was feeling my fear and confusion. As we looked down at our "sought after" baby, he very softly said, "Do you want to know something good about this?" I remember thinking, *Yes, yes, please tell me something good.* He continued, "What I have here is a fishing partner for life." That night, as the three of us cuddled together, a bonding that I will treasure forever began, and continues to grow today.

We were not home with our "bundle" long before my daughter became quite the mother. Ashley had tried to mold and instruct her brother, Tripp, with little success. Trampus was like a little doll that would comply with her every wish. She was in heaven! What would her reaction be when we had to tell her that he was different and that we weren't even sure in what way? But she, like her father, responded as if to say, "What's the problem?" She had fallen in love and nothing and no one could steal that love! One more hurdle we had overcome!

Our eight-year-old son, Tripp, was less intent on the baby and was pretty much coming and going in his own little world, as do eight-year-olds. Although I wasn't sure how much he already knew or how much he could really understand, within a couple of months we decided it was time to sit down and give as much information as he wanted. His young eyes seemed to soften as he listened to my explanation. His first response was, "Is he going to be all right?" I assured him that he was going to be fine and that with all of our help, he was going to be everything God intended him to be. His expression lit up—one of determination and authority. "Well," he said, "they better not give him a hard time or they'll answer to me." Here was Trampus's "protector."

Things were slowly but surely falling into place. The last hurdle—the grandparents. *Ugh*, every time I even thought about it, I would get weak. Their words kept echoing in my mind: *Are you sure you want to start over again? Why are you having a baby this late in life? Why would you want to be tied down again now that the other two are more on their own?* They hadn't even mentioned birth defects or sickness. How would they react to the news since they were already having difficulty with the thought of a so-called "normal" child? Although I know it was very difficult and they had to deal with it each in their own way, they showed nothing but love and acceptance and were captured by our "new bundle." To this day, I am sure my ninety-eight-year-old mother-in-law's motivation to live is because of her best friend and grandson Trampus. He takes pleasure in helping to take care of her, and her pleasure comes in taking care of him. You can't separate them.

The word had pretty much been spread throughout the community, so we really didn't have to make any formal announcements. Each friend in his and her own way offered love and support and helped us to begin our new journey of bringing up a little one who was categorized before he even stepped up to be!

As I processed all that was happening—all the information coming to me—much to my amazement, the only negative thing I could see or feel was related to the outside world's reaction and all the things they said this baby with DS would not be able to do! My thoughts began, *How can they know? They've never been with him; they've never even seen him. How can they be so opinionated? How do they know today what he will or will not do tomorrow, next week or even next year?* As a result of these thoughts, Vince and I made a decision that we would not research the effects of the extra chromosome, but rather would raise him as much like our other two as we could. We decided we would push and encourage Trampus just as we had done with Ashley and Tripp, and if and when we saw him becoming frustrated, we would take a different course.

The most important thing that I believed he needed was to know that he was loved. He was teaching me all about unconditional acceptance. I knew it would be imperative for him to be confident in who he was regardless of how he looked, regardless of his intellectual competence, and regardless of how others felt about his role in our society. I knew he had a purpose, and I was going to give my all in allowing him to not only discover that purpose, but to accomplish it! It is an ongoing battle, but I keep reminding myself that we have the victory, and we continue to press on—one day at a time!

Although I knew Trampus would need lots of attention, he actually demanded very little. He rarely cried and was content wherever we put him. As I worked with him, the thought would come, *Look at him. He's not sitting up yet; he doesn't look like you or anyone else in your family.* People are always staring and seeing that he's different! It was decision time! Do I continue to think these thoughts, or do I go deeper—to the inner man and compare what is already there and what has already been experienced? Every time I have continued to think on those thoughts projected by the world, I have had a piece of my joy stolen; a part of what this baby has for me is taken away. I am then unable to give him the proper encouragement and unconditional love he needs in order to accomplish what he has been created to do. But when I let go of those thoughts and go deep inside and remember what I already know to be the real truth, what a joy he is to work with; how he seems to look in my eyes and say thank you. I am able to enjoy not only the feeling of accomplishment, but receive the never-ending love he has for me to become the person I was created to be!

We lose the joy of raising our children when we allow the world to dictate what our children should desire. We need to be quiet long enough to hear them speak their hearts desire.

As I watched him develop the first few months, I could see that his muscle tone would be a problem and could, in turn, affect his motor skills. I knew for sure we would need to build muscle. Although at this point, my expertise in exercising was within, I was ready to take that energy and desire and put it to work in the outward arena. I was able to find a little mat with a ball, pillows, and a video to help develop an infant. Just what I needed! Suddenly, what we were doing out of necessity became the "in" thing to do—aerobics. I "kinda" like to think we started the trend. I actually developed a timesheet that I would use to schedule his exercise time. We would work on the mat approximately thirty minutes at a time, two to three times a day. I would put him on his stomach on top of the ball, roll him toward me, and then roll him away. Laying him on his back, I would take each arm and spread them to the side, bring them back together, lift them over his head, then bring them down by his side. I would put him on his stomach and lie down in the same position in front of him and try to get his attention in an effort to encourage him to raise his head. Another way of strengthening his neck muscle was to sit him on my hip facing away from me. At first, I would have to hold his chin in my hand, but eventually he could hold it up himself; he would want to look up to follow the sounds and actions around him.

Anything I could think of that would stimulate his body, we did. This was a very important part of his development because I could see that there was no real desire on his part to move about. I began to realize that one of our biggest roles would be to help him learn to desire each thing that most people experience naturally. I would need to become his motivator.

Because I have always loved music, I was always looking for and buying tapes that we could listen to and sing along. He would go to sleep both at naptime and bedtime listening to his tapes.

Another important role that I knew we would play in Trampus's life was to be a mediator between him and the world. We would need to take our learning experiences and reveal them through our lives in the community. This would prove to be one of the most difficult times for me and required the most strenuous parts of my faith exercise program. The part of me that wanted to protect us from the stares, the comments, the unnecessary pity, would rise up, and every time the opportunity came to bring him with us, my feelings would say, *Oh, don't bother to take him to Tripp's ballgame, he'll be better off staying home, he'll get too tired.* I'd come up with excuse after excuse, but I knew in my "inner man" he needed to be a part of everyone's life, and they needed to see and learn all that he could offer. The only way that could happen was for them to be with him. Thank goodness God's desire for him in me is greater than my desire for me!

SIX MONTHS

Within six months, he was sitting up. Much to the surprise and frustration of other mothers with children his age, our little one was patty-caking while his peers sat and stared with envy! Ahhhh, we had overcome another hurdle. We later found out he was not expected to sit up until at least nine to maybe even twelve months. *Oops*—we didn't know! This better explains the difference in information that can come to us from outside, versus the information and desire that is placed within us. We need to learn to go within to meet the needs of those around us. When we can learn to do this, then we are better able to allow the outside information to work for us in a positive way. The God who created every unique individual knows the needs of each and will use us to meet those needs. Had we known and taken the information suggesting he may not sit up until later, would we have tried to encourage him early? I doubt it.

Within a month or two, we began to see what appeared to be his first tooth. Just one problem—it wasn't just one and they were not his front teeth, they were his eyeteeth. Oh great, Dracula in our midst. But, through the mercy of God, the front, top, and bottom soon joined in and all was well.

We didn't encourage crawling, probably because I couldn't figure out how to teach him; but because of his desire to go places, he initiated the effort on his own. He took on the appearance of a crab since he would use only one leg as the moving force dragging along the other. We later were told that he was using one side of his brain and that it would be to his advantage for us to work with him in learning to use both legs. You could tell he was pleased that he now had some say in his going and coming.

The most difficult of the early times with Trampus came as a result of the respiratory problems he began to develop. He seemed susceptible to colds and was not strong enough to fight them off, allowing infection to come from the remaining mucus. The majority of the time, we fought it with antibiotics, although deep down I knew we were putting a Band-Aid on the hurt rather than curing it. I always felt the key was to dry up the mucus. Apparently, it's more complicated for a small child because we were unable to use a decongestant strong enough. The most frustrating thing was the discomfort it caused which would steal his energy and desire. We both needed our strength and energy to fight not only the normal obstacles, but also those that we allowed to manifest that weren't even necessary: concern over perception from the outside world. That shouldn't be an issue.

Although the infections and respiratory problems were very frustrating and pulled a great deal of energy from us, I have to confess that it required time aside from work and accomplishment and allowed time to just be together to hold, nurture, and to love. Too many times, as I look back, I was a "woman with a mission," out to prove, determined to cause the world to look through different eyes! This is not bad in itself, but if we are not careful, it becomes the motivation rather than the results. My real mission is to raise this child so that he will be able to do all that is in his heart to do; to help open doors that might otherwise be shut, and to encourage him even when everything around him tells him to "forget it," or "give it up." There were times when others thought maybe I was babying him too much—rocking him to sleep at night. Somehow deep in my heart, I know those were the times we were communicating when there was no verbal ability to do so. When I would rock him and look in his little eyes, I could so much easier say, "I love you, little one, and more importantly, God loves you. You are so special and you are helping Mommy see life so much clearer." I could give him an extra squeeze, a touch to express what so much of the time I felt was locked up and not able to be verbalized.

We found as we came out of a season where there would seem to be more problems, we would be ready to "charge in" with a new motivation, new strength, and a willingness to learn and grow. Much of this was a result of that inner strength, caring doctors, dear friends and family, and a community that was open to learn.

TODDLER

We celebrated Trampus's first birthday in Columbia with his grandparents. Each member had broken through the barriers of fear and confusion and were truly able to enjoy his precious "ways." He would give a smile that would reach all the way to your toes and bring up things you weren't even aware were in you: joy, peace, appreciation, but most importantly, unconditional love. He would love you with every part of his being no matter what you said or did. I can remember being furious at something his daddy or sister would say. Ready to let them have it with both barrels, he would catch my eye with a look that caused me to stop and consider my reaction to the situation. I would try and reconcile differences with added patience and compassion. I was amazed that he was already accomplishing one of his purposes at the young age of one—exposing the love and forgiveness of his Creator.

Trampus gave us the thrill we had been waiting for with great expectation when he took his first step at sixteen months. He was now independent and could be in charge of his mobility. He had risen to the acclaimed world of the "toddlers," and we were proud of his success as well. For us to watch him work so hard for something that generally comes so easily, continues to help us appreciate those accomplishments.

By the time Trampus was two, we were better prepared financially to begin looking at ways in which we wanted to include the outside world in his day-to-day life: speech therapists, intervention programs, surgeries. We had heard of a medical center in Dallas that would do an overall physical on children with Down syndrome and make recommendations based on the results of those assessments. We spent his second birthday at the center, and Trampus went through a number of physical and psychological tests.

We were told that his hearing, sight, and overall physical health was good. Recommendations were offered concerning speech and the availability of facial surgery in the future to remove any possible discrimination that may occur. They told us about a doctor in Florida that recommended vitamin therapy for Down's children. After visiting the clinic and reviewing the material, we decided that there was no need for any cosmetic surgery, but that we would pursue the vitamins. I'm not sure what part the vitamins played if any since we cannot compare that age without them, but we did come to a place where we questioned its value and stopped the therapy.

We also learned about an organization called The National Association for Child Development (NACD.org). They were wonderful and I recommend their program to anyone interested. Bob Doman, the founder of the program, believes you can teach the mentally disabled, the learning disabled, etc., and works with the parents in developing a program to help overcome the deficiencies of their individual child. The program is reviewed and updated on a quarterly basis. Trampus and I committed as much as four hours a day to the program with the support and help of the other members of the family. We had physical therapy workouts such as walking up and down the stairs for five minutes or what seemed like all day at the time. There were leg bends, weight lifting, even running up and down the sand dunes; all in hopes of strengthening his muscular tone. At the recommendation of NACD, Vince built a stand that formed a thirty-degree triangle. We attached a pair of his shoes, one on each side of the board. I would put Trampus's feet in the shoes, hold his hand, and help him stand and squat. We would do several repetitions at a time.

We learned the tongue was a muscle and that exercising it should be a daily practice. One of the most difficult tasks we had to do was to thump his tongue. This would help prevent his allowing it to protrude. If it was in fact a muscle, then he could learn to strengthen it in order to control it. It was heartbreaking to see the expression on his face each time we had to correct him. The need for this exercise diminished as he became conscious of his tongue in his mouth. The only time we really noticed this issue was when he was overly tired. Even today, in those seldom circumstances, the minute our eyes meet and I show some sign of mouth movement, he immediately gets control.

Along with the tongue exercises, there were visual workouts which included flashcard games. I began to use flash cards with the alphabet on them and we would sound out each letter. Because he has such a good memory, he was able to retain the letter and the sound it made. Later, when he began to read, he would sound out the words. This would allow him to "figure out" some of the words that he didn't know. This is still a valuable tool in his reading. I was told that children with DS were unable to learn with phonics. They supposedly learn through memorization of words. I believe there is a place for both and am glad that we used the same method on him as we did with his sister and brother.

I would take strong smells and introduce them to him, identifying the smell, i.e., onions, roses, etc. This would help stimulate his sense of smell. In the same way, I would sensitize his sensory perception of touch by putting his hands in ice-cold water and then warm water specifying "warm" and "cold" with each exposure. We would play guessing games with food by covering his eyes and having him identify different foods distinguishing between spicy, sweet, sour, etc.

One important bit of information was that the oxygen that goes to the brain through the nose is more effective than through the mouth. Many times I would just use my hand over his mouth and we would play a game of how many times he could "sniff" before I let go.

The most important thing to me was to see him as a computer. You can't ask anything back from the computer until you have programmed it. Don't get angry with the computer if it takes longer to program. Just keep feeding the information in, and in time, you will begin to get it back. When you feed information into the brain, you are stimulating and producing a foundation on which to build. I'm sure that was what was happening, although his understanding was not always apparent. We would put puzzles together and play sequencing games, but the one thing I did probably more than anything else was just read to him. We would carry his books everywhere we went. There are so many lessons to be learned in that one theory. This confirmed for me the importance of what I was putting into my own mind—unfair expectations and demands based on my own selfish desires for accomplishment. I was taking in the world's conclusion of what Trampus could and couldn't do. I was letting the world dictate to me, rather than just providing the nurturing and the information he needed and required according to his time frame.

He was now actively a part of the family and we began to focus on his behavior as such. It was important for him to begin to learn what was acceptable and what was not. We have always been firm believers that each of us must carry his/her own load and must abide by the rules set for the family unit. Although it has required patience and perseverance, we continue to keep this at the top of our "need" list for him.

PRESCHOOL

I could sense from my husband that it was just a matter of time before he was going to insist that I release our gift into the world. Send him out into the world to learn and experience others? It was too early, he was too young, and I didn't want him to learn about the world. After all, hadn't I finally come to the decision that the only problems I had was with the *world*? We were doing great without it! I had learned, however, that God had given me Vince with incredible insight and wisdom. Since this was a walk of faith, I knew I needed to listen.

Trampus did need my love and nurturing and protection, but he also needed the world to help test his decisions, offer goals and reasons to pick and choose what he wanted to learn.

One incident I remember that confirmed the importance of including these special children in the lives of others came when Trampus was very young. It involved a neighbor that lived across the side street from our house. Bennie was in our Bible study group, so Trampus would see her often. She also had a German Shepherd that she walked past the house each day on their way to the beach.

We began to have trouble with Trampus staying indoors. Although we lived in a community that for the most part was gated, our house was on the beach side so we were not. If anyone left a door cracked or if the door could be easily opened, he would quietly scoot out to investigate the world. All of the bedrooms, with the exception of one, had access to the outside decks. We tried to be conscious of keeping doors locked; however, a time came when the one leading out of Trampus's room was not. It was a combination glass/screen door and for some reason if the door slammed shut, it would automatically lock.

It was around November. The weather was cold and we had all gone to bed. I remember hearing a ringing and trying to get my bearings as I heard Vince say hello. My heart stopped as I listened for some clue as to the caller. It was 5:00 a.m. and I heard Vince say, "Yes, ma'am, thank you so much, we're on our way." It seems Trampus's door was not locked; he woke up and decided to venture out. We believe that when he went out, the door slammed and locked, so he couldn't get back in. I think the bell for our doors were very high, but even if he had pushed them, I don't think we could have heard them in our bedroom upstairs. We were all amazed at his ability to remember our neighbor and to go to her (he was able to reach her doorbell) and wake her up. He told her he couldn't get in the house, so naturally she scooped him up and brought him inside to get him warm. She said her first thought was that something terrible had happened to our entire family. Although it was a horribly frightening experience, after the fact, we were thankful that Trampus's connection to others provided him an opportunity to get help when he needed it.

After finally accepting that his community and peers could help him learn—help provide him a picture to copy—I began the phone calls to see who wanted to benefit from our precious package.

It was during this time I learned a wonderful lesson. Just because you believe something—that doesn't make it "truth." People make decisions based on programming from our society. If they are not open for new information, then the decision may come that would steal a wonderful experience from them. I believe that has happened throughout the lives of many who have had an opportunity to be exposed to Trampus but have believed they weren't "equipped."

One local privately owned daycare and preschool informed me they were not able to handle a child with Down syndrome even though they admitted to knowing nothing about it. I started to argue and to persuade them they were wrong, but I got a "check" with my inner man. *Oh well, their loss!* Because my family had very little exposure to early child care, I knew finding a place for Trampus would be a challenge.

The next call was a soft-spoken woman who quietly listened as I explained our hopes for our little toddler. Her response was, "Well, we've never had a child with DS and so we really don't know anything about it." I offered my well-thought-out response, "And I'm glad. We don't either. We just keep exposing him the same way we did our other two children. When something becomes too difficult or too confusing for Trampus, we back away." After a tour of the facilities, all parties were in agreement that Trampus would become a daycare student at Woodland Hall. Thank you, Julie Hiott and Kristen Zeaser-Sydow for opening your doors and hearts allowing Trampus to be a part of what you worked so hard to provide for our young children!

We had succeeded over the first hurdle. He was accepted and wanted in an environment that would offer good role modeling. Woodland Hall was known for their structure and discipline—a perfect environment for our little "piece of clay."

The memories of those next two years are wonderful. Trampus was potty-trained within a few months. He had watched the other children go to the potty and just as we suspected, he then wanted to do the same. They had programs available such as Kindermusic, Jumpnastics, and even ballet. They would come in to work with the children if the parents were interested. Trampus loved his music and worked hard at his tumbling!

One very special memory for me—and I believe for the school and teachers too—came when I decided I wanted to sign him up for drama. One of the wonderful gifts he has is that he loves to entertain, to perform. I had decided it was important to watch for things he did well and enjoyed.

I'll never forget the somewhat fearful look on Lori Carroll's face (she worked with children interested in drama and amazingly ended up teaching him while he was a student at Wando High School). It seemed her expression was telling me, "She is asking too much this time. She's expecting too much from us and him." Thankfully, my power of persuasion helped her to relinquish her preconceived ideas and she accepted Trampus into the program. They were going to perform as a touring circus show. Trampus would be a juggling clown. As the day of the performance arrived, the excitement was building. Each performer was appropriately dressed and the announcement was made: "The Circus has come to town!" The spotlight fell on the lion tamer, a young boy with a stick, which he proceeded to use to draw on the floor while keeping his face focused on the ground with little action. The spotlight traveled on to the ballerina who was looking beautiful in her tutu; unfortunately, she too was mesmerized by the floor and refused to perform her well-practiced routine. Well, the spotlight found its way to the last hope of a successful show—the juggling clown. At this point my heart was fluttering, but I knew my little performer was truly getting ready to do what he loved without any concern for those around him. He loved to do what was being asked and never thought whether or not anyone would be pleased. He had practiced and he was ready! When those little hands came up pretending to throw balls up and down and that grin of satisfaction went across that little face, I do not remember when I have been happier for the success of someone else. Lori's eyes met mine, and although it was difficult for us to see each other through our tears, we knew we had both learned a beautiful lesson. Always pursue the desire in your heart and don't ever let your mind stop you from allowing an opportunity to do something you may think is not feasible.

While our toddler's experiences at Woodland Hall were wonderful, we heard about the Montessori School West of the Ashley and that they accepted children with DS. Here was an opportunity to expose him to academics based on desire. One of the problems I've learned about Trampus is that there are no established desires. Just as he had to learn to want to go potty or learn his own name, or learn the need to eat, he also had to desire to "want" to play and "to learn." That is where "role modeling" or "peer participation" is so important for children with Down syndrome. Being able to be with children younger and older in the Montessori environment gave him confidence. The success of doing what the younger children could not do, while the older students stimulated a desire to do what he couldn't do, as he watched them was invaluable. I have always believed the best tool for learning is experiencing it. We see the proof in our everyday lives. If I read the instructions for an activity; I may say that I know how to do it, but until I put action to the words, there is no assurance I can accomplish it. This has been a great reminder for me as I live out my faith. I can see that my faith, without working it out, has little effect on my life and the lives around me. However, when I take what I learn through the Scriptures and put them to practice, not only do I benefit from them in my own life, but it produces better relationships and I'm able to offer more encouragement and help in the lives of those around me.

The most difficult thing for Trampus to adjust to in Montessori school was the independent work. I've always been there to guide him all of his life, so he expected that same help. It was a wonderful time for Trampus and for us, and we might still be there except for something that happened in the grocery store in Mt. Pleasant. Trampus was not yet four. It was around January and he was helping select several fruits from the stand. Suddenly, we heard this voice "Are you Trampus Hoover?" We had grown accustomed to young children and familiar faced parents speaking, but I knew I had never even seen this person.

After acknowledging that he was in fact Trampus, this lovely lady introduced herself. Probably the foundation of all of our school success, she was the Early Childhood Development (ECD) teacher at Whitesides Elementary School—Mary Meehan. She explained a little bit about the program and helped me get connected to the right people that would get Trampus involved.

PRESCHOOL/KINDERGARTEN

Naturally, since our other two children attended Catholic schools, we began the process of trying to enroll Trampus in kindergarten. (This was prior to meeting Mary Meehan). What a crushing blow to hear that he would not be able to be a part of the educational community of our Parish. After all the many requests for funding for the Catholic school was noted as being for "all" of God's children. It was very difficult to hear that they were not "equipped" to handle a child with special needs. *Ouch!* Our community of faith was lost when it came to handling a child of God who probably needed them more than the so-called "normal" child.

After several meetings with those in the decision-making process, the final proclamation was that Trampus would not be able to attend our local Catholic school. They would, however, form a committee to research how to "handle" these children. Our question, of course, was "what shall we do in the meantime?"

Initially, we were devastated. Vince wrote a very demonstrative letter to the bishop. Unfortunately, we never received a reply from the bishop. We did receive a letter from the pastor of our Parish expressing his embarrassment concerning our letter to the bishop. It seemed our letter did not accomplish its purpose, but rather stirred up controversy between us and the hierarchy. The appearance was there was more concern over "feelings" than what might be best for our son. I was really confused as to why the church would take a stand against abortion of these special need children, yet they were comfortable with rejecting them in their programs. All of a sudden, I had a new appreciation for our Heavenly Father's suffering over the rejection of His son. Obviously, they just "didn't get it." We tried for a while to agree to disagree. Unfortunately, the resentment we were harboring became too strong.

Vince eventually determined that he could not continue to be a part of what he saw as hypocrisy, so we made the difficult decision to come out of the organized church. I have to admit there were times I questioned that decision, but the most important thing I had learned from my guide book, "The Word of God," was that the two of us needed to be one and God had set up His system with one head for the family—the husband. As a result of our experience, we remained out of the "church" environment for almost a decade. Thank goodness our relationship with our "Creator" is not founded on "church," but rather a personal relationship with Him. The fellowship of a church body is important and with God's help, we have been able to return to the Eucharist.

My prayer will continue to go up for those who have the responsibility of making decisions for *all* Catholic schools. They must see that inclusion is a very real and successful option in the academics of the faith community. We are supposed to see ourselves as "the body of Christ," so it is very important to acknowledge each of its parts. They must embrace all of God's children and allow them to be involved in all aspects of the life of the church.

Because of God's grace and desire to take what the enemy intends for bad and work it for good, a door opened for us that has provided Trampus with what I believe has been the best exposure he could have ever gotten. I believe, at this point, it is imperative that I stress the fact that God is not a respecter of persons; what He does for me, He's waiting and wanting to do for anyone who will call on Him. It is faith that pleases God; not doing the right thing, but believing He will direct our paths and help when we don't know what to do or where to go.

Enter Mary Meehan. Because of her involvement and her prayers and expectations, Trampus began an academic and social experience that has allowed him to participate in any event he has desired. Her encouragement and support to each teacher that agreed to have him in his/her class provided him the opportunity to prove Mary right.

While academics have always been important to us, I must continue to stress that it was and is not our emphasis for Trampus. Having the ability to look back, I believe my communicating that fact helped keep doors open with Trampus's teachers. Because we believed his greatest need was to be able to be a part of the whole; we refused the temptation of the educational community to focus on his language and math skills. We understood and still understand their desire to increase the knowledge of their students, but we also believe that the intellectually gifted will receive that knowledge. When given time and patience, Trampus continued to increase in those skills also. There is, at the same time, however, another form of education needed that may be more important: how to function together by taking all of that knowledge and producing a society that is not dysfunctional; one that flows together, building itself up in love and concern for all mankind. This type of education would teach humility as well as respect for authority.

If you run a business, you need an accountant or a computer system that has the capabilities of computing payroll taxes, warehousing inventory, etc. But as important as that sophisticated system is, I suggest that you don't need that expensive system just to keep a record of your personal checking account. All that is really needed is a simple adding machine. If, however, you do not keep good records on that simple checking account, there will be no need for the business side. Do we think of the adding machine as disabled or not useable because of its simplicity? I think not. There is an important role for both. Since society is made up of every unique individual, it is to the advantage of all to find and allow each member to take his or her place.

Because we came into the program late, we decided to let him continue in the ECD program the following year. This gave him time to mature and practice learning in a corporate environment.

The only problem that I could see with ECD was lack of time. The program was from 8:20 until 11:20. He was ready for a longer schedule, and I knew he would flourish with the extra help. He needed to experience learning without an adult by his side.

Once again, Woodland Hall came to my mind; only now it would be the kindergarten program, not just day care. I was so excited about the revelation that he could go to Whiteside's in the morning and Woodland Hall after lunch.

Needless to say, I was surprised when I went to enroll him and heard them saying "Martha, can he stay quietly in his seat? Can he learn in a structured environment?" I could hear the fear and negativism, but the one thing I had learned was that all issues had to be resolved openly and properly. I explained with as much compassion as I could muster, but with authority that rose up from inside me, "Trampus has proven that he is capable of learning but I'm particularly impressed that your five-year-olds *all* stay in their seats!" I saw a look come over her face and before she had a chance to respond, I continued, "I don't have a problem with your telling me that Woodland Hall doesn't know how to teach Trampus, but when we leave, it will be your problem in teaching—not Trampus's problem learning."

She asked for a little time to think about it and called back a day or two later to tell me they would love to have Trampus in their kindergarten program. A very important thing I have learned: make sure he's wanted and not being forced on anyone, and let the final decision be theirs! When they make the decision, it becomes their success as well as his. I always make an exerted effort to remove the burden of his success from their teaching skills, and place the burden on his desire to learn what they are offering. If he is interested and wants it after being exposed to it, then he will participate in the learning process. If not, it doesn't matter how well they teach—he won't receive it.

Fortunately, my husband and I believe strongly in discipline, because I am convinced that discipline has been one of the major contributing factors in allowing Trampus to be involved in community and school activities. Although he may have difficulty in receiving information and then expressing the same, he could and can understand "yes" and "no." He has always been very determined, and we have to make a decision to stand firm when necessary regardless of his reaction.

I might add, that the determination within him has been the tool that has brought him many victories; but had we not helped guide that determination, I believe he would have been forced many times to remain on the outside looking in. It takes a tremendous constitution to hold firm when you face these trials or tests. Again, I am thankful that Vince saw the need to do so. When I wanted to waiver, or just tire from the confrontations, he would remind me that it was for Trampus and that we really had no choice. I remember one particular time that was very difficult for me to watch. We were in Mass and Trampus would not remain seated and quiet. His dad very assuredly stood up, proceeded to march him out right down the middle aisle of the church. *Ugh!* Really, down the middle for all to see? I'm not sure what happened that morning in the front of the church, but his dad never had to initiate the march again. Today, as a result of consistency when he was young, our confrontations are minimal and always end with his compliance, and very quickly he's back to his smiling, agreeable self.

An important motivation for me in the discipline area is the fact that everyone can be trained; training does not require intellect. We can even train our animals. The Scripture that confirms this for me is found in Proverbs 22:6 (NKJV), "Train-up a child in the way he should go, and when he is old he will not turn from it." It is interesting to me that we are not instructed to "educate" in the way they should go. Again, while some may not be educable, all can be trained. This should better persuade each of us to put education in its proper place, following the most important requirement—training.

Very seldom have I had to use my hand on Trampus's behind, but I would do so when he refused to listen. We would not accept his decision to disobey, and if I questioned his ability to understand, we talked about it after the spanking. He eventually learned that I was not going to accept his disobedience, and that if we had to remove him from doing what he wanted to do, we would. We refused to handle his behavior any differently from that of his sister and brother regardless of his understanding. I'm convinced that there were many times my other children didn't understand our discipline, but it didn't stop me from being firm with what I knew was right. Trampus will respond quickly for others when the threat of contacting us is presented to him.

No one, child or adult, wants to be responsible for making decisions until they are equipped to do so, thus, the reason for parenting our children. They grow up understanding the consequences of bad choices and begin to back away from decisions that can cause pain. This is true of everyone, regardless of ability or social circumstances.

One of the blessings we received, while Trampus was still young, was a beautiful little granddaughter named Emily. Ashley had married her childhood sweetheart and they were parenting while going to the University of South Carolina (USC). Since she was so precious and incredibly smart, it was not long before she was a perfect "best friend" to her uncle, and has continued to be a wonderful teacher and supporter. (Now there are four more adorable grandchildren in the Bolchoz family—Daniel, Elizabeth, Vincent and Manning—as well as Tripp's three precious "Hoover grands," Andrew, Eliza, and Caroline. Each one plays a tremendous role in the development of their Uncle Trampus.)

ELEMENTARY SCHOOL

The day arrived when we had to present our little man to the real thing—five-year kindergarten. Mary had handpicked the teacher, and she took over what Mary was no longer in a position to continue. This gifted lady was Susie Benton. She stepped in and brought Trampus into the world of twenty-two other young people, rather than the eight he had grown to love. We were able to keep some ties with Mary because Trampus was taking Taekwondo from her. Her patience and ability to not only teach, but also stimulate the desire to learn, brought Trampus to the green belt level. Unfortunately, the sequencing became more difficult and because it took longer for him to progress to the next level, he became discouraged and frustrated. I'm not sure we made the right decision in allowing him to quit, but you have to choose your battles and time becomes important if you're going to pursue different ventures. He has to want it badly enough to put forth the extraordinary effort he needs to succeed.

Susie, with Mary's help, became Trampus's advocate. There are so many fun stories about his kindergarten years, but one that I loved was when Susie informed me that it was important for Trampus to know his full name. *Ouch!* Payback time. (I knew we should have just named him Bill.) Unfortunately, the same time that I was trying to get him to repeat "William Sunday Trampus Hoover," Susie was teaching him the days of the week. So, here we would go—William Sunday Monday Tuesday…uh oh… competition with information. I finally came up with a solution. We gave each finger on his hand a name, i.e., the thumb was William, the pointer was Sunday, the middle was Trampus, and the ring finger was Hoover. Every time he would start to say his name, he would lift each finger. When he would finish with Sunday and want to repeat Monday, he would lift up that middle finger and remember its name was Trampus. Yea! We overcame probably one of the biggest battles Vince and I alone created.

We were told that in order to determine Trampus's academic needs, it would be necessary for him to be tested. We were advised to have that testing done by an outside psychologist rather than the one used by the schools. They felt this would give him the best advantage to present the most desirable case for inclusion. Trampus and I had spent an incredible amount of time reading books, looking at flash cards of birds, bugs, and all kinds of "critters." He could identify a variety of insects. I'll never forget when the testing was over and the psychologist began to go over the results. I was amazed at some of the criteria used to determine his IQ. We went head to head when it became evident that the fact that he couldn't identify an umbrella would have an impact on the final outcome. As I pointed out to the psychologist, "You are going to determine how smart he is by whether or not he knows what you know? I don't use an umbrella and have never exposed him to one, but I wonder…would she be able to identify a monarch butterfly or an earwig bug? Oh well, as far as I was concerned, we had proven he could learn. Now we had to expose him to what society deemed essential for him to know.

Because of the atmosphere of love and commitment to each child at Mamie Whitesides Elementary, Trampus became a successful forerunner for inclusion. Principal Dave Schlacter and Assistant Principal Lona Pounder remained open the entire time Trampus was at Whitesides, and provided all the support needed both for us and his teachers which allowed inclusion to succeed.

I have always felt that I know what is best for Trampus, and many times have had to fight the emotions that wanted to override someone else's intervention. Thank goodness I have learned to be quiet first and take time to re-evaluate circumstances before stepping in.

One important lesson that I believe needed to be learned involved independence. Trampus's first grade teacher, while very compassionate and caring, did not pamper the children or do things for them. I would volunteer to help with field trips and was amazed the way she expected the children to keep up. Very quickly they all realized they had to follow her. I guess I was afraid they wouldn't, so I was constantly trying to "herd" them. I still marvel at how she was able to know when to look back and just how long to allow them to "catch up" and find her. Needless to say, as I saw them do more and more on their own, I would give Trampus space and time to do it without me. By learning responsibility, at whatever level, Trampus has been able to participate with less intervention. Now, if there is a need to be responsible for something issued to him, he will make the effort to keep up with it. (I had to purchase several library books in the process of learning this lesson, but now he keeps up with his phone, wallet, etc., and the effort we put forth when he was young has made it much easier as he has gotten older.)

As far as I know, each teacher that has had Trampus in his/her class made that decision on their own, and I can honestly say that each one has reported nothing but joy in having him.

A funny classroom story while Trampus was at Whitesides once again included music. As mentioned before, we were always listening to music and looking for fun musical instruments. It was one thing that I loved, and he seemed to respond to it with great enthusiasm. I think he was in the first grade when I found the cutest violin that had music recorded in it. You could select from several songs and when the instrument was on, every time you ran the bow over the strings, it would play out the song one note at a time. His favorite tune was "Ode to Joy." He informed me one morning that he was going to take it to school for "show" day and play for everyone. Astonishment from the class led to "how on earth was Trampus capable of playing that violin." We all still laugh out loud when we remember the eyes of both teacher and students as the song would slowly play each note perfectly as he ran the bow over the strings.

Trampus's elementary school years passed with very few battles. Sometimes I would have to remind the school that the expectations, even in his behavior, required some space and patience. I would have to remind them that sometimes they needed to back off and get the microscope off of him. They would naturally tend to be too demanding both of him and me in the beginning. When I pointed this out in kindness, they always would be able to see it and back off. Things would then seem to line back up. One example was when Mrs. Benton called me in to discuss Trampus's behavior during circle time in the mornings. Of course we had a firm discussion on obedience or the possibility of removal from the class. Unfortunately, I got another call and then another. Finally, I realized I needed to back off and evaluate the situation. Sometimes we get caught up in defending authority rather than researching the problem. I decided to bring out a point of behavior by asking if Trampus was the only one that seemed to be causing trouble in the circle. I think it wasn't until then that Mrs. Benton realized that maybe because she had such an easy access to me as well as my willingness to help, she was requiring more from us than others. Certainly other children were being disobedient at times, but she wasn't always able to get help from their parents. I also had had time to think about his actions and offered the probability that he had found a way to force his removal from an activity he didn't particularly enjoy.

Another incident I remember involved the principal. It happened when attention was being drawn to behavior problems in the schools. Violence had become an issue, so the faculty and staff were sensitive to the students' actions. We think Trampus had found an old pocket knife of his grandfather's and decided to bring it to school to show it off.

I remember the call from Principal Dave Schlacter. He asked if I could come by the school for a conference. *Uh-oh!* He mentioned the knife. My stomach was churning the whole way to the school. What had he done and what would they do? When I arrived at the office, one of the secretaries smiled at me and offered to get Dave. (Such a small world. That same sweet lady, Shirley Low, is now the "other" grandmommy to my precious "Hoover" grands!) By the time he came out of his office, I was just about in tears. He asked me to step into his office and asked Trampus to wait outside. As we passed each other, Trampus looked up and said "Hi, Mom!" with a big smile and walked right on by me.

Dave smiled and apologized for my unscheduled appointment. He explained that they had decided that it was best for Trampus to realize the "error of his ways" by sending him to the principal's office. Dave began to tell me what happened after that. He started his story with a bit of a laugh and explained that what began as a session for discipline had quickly become a question and answer period between him and Trampus; Trampus was the interrogator. Dave had started to reprimand him and Trampus wanted to know who the people were in the picture on Dave's desk. Dave said before it was over, he felt like Trampus knew more about him than most. He did say he thought he had gotten through to Trampus that he should never bring his pocketknife to school again, but it was the most unique discipline encounter with a student he had ever experienced.

Because I believe it is important to help the people who are willing to include Trampus, I have made it a point to be available as much as possible.

When Trampus was younger, there were times when I would be told by a teacher or staff member of a situation brewing between Trampus and another child. As I tried to investigate before I intervened, I would find that many times the other student was unaware of Trampus's differences. Usually, I would be able to find the opportunity to take that child off to the side and explain how important their interaction was with Trampus and how much I appreciated patience with him. I tried—and still do at times—to help them to understand by explaining that when Trampus was born, some of the areas that allow us to learn and do things did not fully develop in him. He would learn slowly some of the things that we learn quickly. I would go on to explain that he can learn many of these things, but it takes him a lot longer, and he needs much more help than most of us. Usually, the other child (and those that deal with Trampus still today) immediately began to see their relationship with Trampus differently, and they would try to teach him and include him with a completely new attitude. People, most of the time, are very kind and considerate if time is taken to help them see things through Trampus's eyes. I have had to learn through trial and error and when possible, I can help others learn too with less frustration for them.

One particular area that I remember required my involvement was in PE. I had always known that my older children were hesitant to try something they weren't confident they could do successfully. They were not quick to try things they didn't understand and didn't feel they could do. Trampus was no different. Since motor skills were his most difficult hurdle, he was less than enthusiastic about the PE class. Everything moved fast and instructions had to be grasped quickly. I began to get little notes expressing concern and frustration from his PE teacher, Ms. Acuff, because he wasn't listening and following instructions. The first thing I did was to sit down with Trampus and to remind him of his responsibility to obey. He had to learn that he had to respect authority, and I would have to remind him that many times we have to work harder to do the things that are difficult for us. Because he loved school so much, I was always able to use that as leverage in getting him to put up with more than he wanted. I would remind him that the alternative to giving up and being disobedient was to stay home.

Next, I went to the teacher and helped her to understand his reasons for being defiant. I explained that it was difficult for him to take in all of the instructions as quickly as the other students. I believed he wanted to be like the other students so badly that he would not risk trying and failing. (For that reason, many times he will still refuse to do something.) We should always remember that when people are dealing with our children, especially for the first time, we must help communicate what we have learned through the benefit of the time we've had with them. Others will usually react to the actions they see without considering any hidden reasons.

I reassured the teacher that it had nothing to do with her or her teaching method, but rather his inability to explain or maybe even understand his own rebellion. I offered to come into the class and help with communication so that he was more confident to try.

She then said she had not realized his confusion and that she would like to work on it without me. She agreed that if she needed me, she would call. She and Trampus became the "best of buddies" and she was probably one of his greatest advocates. He thoroughly enjoyed his PE through the entire elementary years and learned many wonderful skills, including the game of soccer. Because the other children saw her patience and success, they were willing to include Trampus in their "recess soccer" so he became very good at the game. He played on the Unified Spirit Soccer Team for Special Olympics South Carolina and passed off the ball to a peer who scored the winning goal at the fall games at Furman University in Greenville, South Carolina. *Yes!*

Mainstreaming, which simply places the child in the classroom with no support, does not work. Inclusion with resource was an alternative that worked for us. I believe with resources provided by the school, coupled with the input of parents knowing their children and offering mediation, inclusion can be successful at the lower levels of education.

Because maturity plays an important role in academic success, we decided to let Trampus repeat the second grade. He had the opportunity to enjoy an extra year in the ECD program, but we decided we could benefit from one more year of delay without any real detriment. As a result, he developed relationships with children one year ahead of him and one year behind him. When we made the move to middle school, he knew many of the seventh graders, which provided some security for him at the new school.

I have discovered that teachers with a natural gift to teach are adequately prepared to instruct children with special needs. The sad thing is many times they don't realize it because they have accepted society's decision that these children must be handled differently, and that information must be gained through education.

I don't mean to imply that it is not necessary to educate teachers concerning children with special needs. I just think we've had too much isolation of special education from regular education. The two environments need to interact particularly at the elementary level. I believe the separation could be the biggest hindrance that exists in preventing not only children with special needs to grow, but also hinders the opportunity for all children to learn about each other. There is a void in learning ways to interact and help each other fill gaps that may exist. Trampus is proof that the unified circumstances in his life have produced the success that he now enjoys. I only regret that I did not have this understanding to give to my other children when they were young.

Each teacher, at one time or another, has shared with me that their experiences with Trampus has increased their ability to interact with the other students as well. One teacher told me about how another child had gotten so excited about Trampus's success in climbing the pole that put him at the top of the "toy fort." She had debated on whether to intervene since the children were encouraging him to climb, and she wasn't sure if he would be able to do it. She watched as one child began to instruct him on putting each hand up and then pulling up, squeezing his legs, and lifting his hands up higher. To her surprise, he followed the instructions and made it to the top. Although Trampus was pleased with his accomplishment, she said it didn't compare with the excitement of the child that came running to her to explain how he had taught Trampus how to climb to the top of the pole. She also mentioned that this classmate was struggling in some areas and it was wonderful seeing him enjoy his success. I love hearing about the experiences from those who have had a chance to interact with Trampus. It's always fun to watch the joy they encounter and the encouragement he is able to give to those who choose to be a part of his life.

Most of his teachers have said that their teaching skills have been sharpened as a result of his presence in their room. One thing we all have agreed on: anything needed over and beyond the normal teaching skills has only benefited the other students; never taken away. I must reiterate again that a very important key in the success of inclusion is appropriate behavior. No one will remove a child from the learning environment as long as they are not disrupting that environment. I also stress the point that there are children with normal learning abilities that can cause disruption and hinder learning. Here we go back to the old "training" which is imperative for all, and a lesson from which our society as a whole could benefit if practiced!

School is a wonderful place for role modeling for all children regardless of their needs. I believe it is particularly important at the elementary level. Many times the educational community is concerned with the effects of having children with special needs in the regular classroom, but Trampus and other children like him have proven that the concern is just not warranted. We felt it was important for Trampus's educational environment to be as normal as possible so we never pushed for an aide to be with him.

While pursuing inclusion for Trampus, I remember visiting our state senator, Arthur Ravenel. I understood he had an adult son with Down syndrome and I wanted to be connected just in case I needed some help. I wanted him on our side. As we talked, I could see the interest but sensed he questioned whether this was attainable. I'll never forget the day he decided to stop by Whitesides to check on Trampus. He wanted to see for himself the results of our quest. It was very exciting for the school and I could tell by watching, he was satisfied with the outcome. We want to thank you, Senator Ravenel, for your willingness to advocate for those in need of a "little help."

Again, as I pointed out earlier, while academics was and is important to us, it has never been our main focus. It will always be necessary for Trampus to be able to interact with others, and we have never felt that it would be accomplished through intellectual success.

I do remember one particular period of time when the school was beginning to question whether or not it was time for him to go into a self-contained classroom. They knew that I felt strongly about inclusion, but they also knew I wanted what was best for all. They had one of the school psychologists test Trampus. They told me about the testing after the fact because the child that was scheduled was absent that day. At first I was upset, but remained silent and remembered that nothing happens without a reason and they were doing what they believed was right. It shouldn't have been that difficult for me to trust their decision because we had already had one wonderful turn of events. Ms. Benton had left the kindergarten class and had taken the position as resource teacher. I like to think she couldn't let go of Trampus. She informed me the results of the test and offered "good news" and "not so good news." I requested the "not so good news" first. She began by explaining that he was given no help whatsoever with the test. As a result, his IQ was determined to be around 50. I remember staring at her and thinking, *How does he put one foot in front of the other? How does he dress himself or feed himself.* Please give me the "good news" quickly! The "good news" was that this school psychologist included in her report that she had never tested a child at this level with as much interaction, eye contact, and communication, and that this was an example of the lack of importance that should be placed on the IQ score. She went on to tell the school that they should keep up with exactly what they were doing, and he should not be put in a self-contained class. I'm sure this testing was allowed in order to dismantle any rationalization when people try to attribute his success to a higher IQ than most children with Down syndrome. I continuously recount this incident because I believe it demonstrates the truth in our philosophy and confirms it with the educational community itself. I didn't have to pay someone to provide a report to support what I wanted and believed to be best for Trampus. Although the report provided the power to keep Trampus included, it was important to remind all those involved that our ultimate goal was what would be "best" for everyone. What we all know is that mainstreaming does not work. If we needed to get help for him in the classroom over and beyond what the teacher could give, then I would pursue it. Since we had not requested an aide for Trampus at this point, all extra help came from his resource teacher.

They assured me that behavior was not a problem, but they had noticed a growing lack of focus. The news I had hoped never to hear was beginning to come forth. Had we considered help through medication? *Ugh!* I always believed it was used to control behavior and so I had avoided it like the plague. They recommended I talk with his doctor about "attention deficit disorder."

When I called his doctor, he told me with compassion that he had believed this was going to be necessary at some point. He believed as the demands on him increased it would become more difficult for him to sustain the level of success he had been enjoying. He recommended that we give him the medication over the weekend and observe any differences. I took his advice, but as of Saturday evening, I saw none. Of course we really weren't doing anything requiring his undivided attention, but I was beginning to believe it was not going to help.

We got up Sunday, I gave him his medicine, and we were off to mass. I took him to the Confraternity of Christian Doctrine (CCD) and purposely said nothing to anyone about the medicine. When I came to pick him up from class, his CCD teacher couldn't get to me fast enough. "Martha, I don't understand it and I can't explain it," she went on, "but Trampus had an incredible day today. He participated in all that we did and seemed to enjoy it more than usual. He stayed on task with the other children." I knew at that point that like it or not, I needed to provide Trampus with all the help available, even if I wasn't completely comfortable with it.

As important as I believe inclusion is at the lower levels of education, it is just as important in other community activities. The more interaction others have with our children and the more our children see and are around other children, the better our society will be as a whole. We will benefit all of our children by allowing them to learn how to become a part of the whole and how to give to the whole.

I always felt the challenge of looking for ways that Trampus could accomplish what was being asked of the other students. I remember when he was asked to write a report on South Carolina. *Yuk!* Write a report. I didn't like to do that when I was in school and could write, so I sure didn't want to do it for someone else. Suddenly, I thought, *Why not record a report. Let him* play *the MC and rather than write, we would visit and talk about the South Carolina facts.* Our project began and we had a ball. We were able to set up an appointment with Senator Ravenel. We traveled to Columbia to meet and see the legislators in action. We visited the Battery, The Yorktown Aircraft Carrier, and Fort Sumter by boat. He interviewed Anne Worsham Richardson, a local artist who was a naturalist and also worked in rehabilitating wild birds. The artist received commendations for her work as a wildlife conservationist from the US Department of the Interior and the US and SC Wildlife Association. She was nominated into the SC Hall of Fame. We actually were amazed when he had completed the project and we had the video put to music. Everyone enjoyed seeing it as much as we did producing it.

We had an opportunity to get involved in the scouts through the Tiger Cubs, but Trampus really got excited when we moved up to the Cub Scouts. I served as assistant leader to the troop so that I would be there to help if needed. He loved the uniform and the awards ceremony where he would receive recognition for his work. He was very serious about the ceremonies and always received a warm applause for his accomplishments. The children were supportive and while I'm sure they realized there were differences, they never saw it more than other differences among themselves. I remember one particular time when one of the TV stations had come to the school to interview Trampus and his teacher in regard to inclusion. The boys had advanced to Webelos Scouts and were on their way to the meeting held in the school library. As they passed the classroom, they saw the TV camera and interviewer talking with the teacher and Trampus. They questioned me as to why Trampus was "getting this attention." I tried to explain that it was related to his learning differences, but I could tell they didn't see any reason regardless of my explanation. They had been with Trampus since they were four and five years old so they had learned to interact with him all of their school lives. They had learned to see the many ways they were alike rather than focusing on the differences.

We stayed involved in scouting. Although the interaction with these friends came through the scouting functions, it at least provided a sense of a social life. These friendships gave him the necessary help to keep up with all of the activities. The meetings allowed Trampus the opportunity to watch the other boys sit and listen to instruction, then move around with the different activities planned.

When it was time to move up to Boy Scouts, our den visited several of the troops. We wanted to find the one that best fit the goals and expectations we had grown to embrace. One of the major deciding factors for us was going to be based on the decision of one of Trampus's closest and dearest friends, Corbin Fuller. Although Corbin and Trampus had only been together in the last year of Webelos, they had been in the same classroom since the second grade. Corbin was not only a wonderful friend, but he proved to be his "protector and teacher" as well. His patience with Trampus was incredible all the way through high school.

After my usual relinquishing of a decision to include God's will and after consulting with the Fullers and his Webelos leader, we became a part of Boy Scout Troop 15. The troop was truly an inspiration and example of an organization teaching young men how to become conscientious, caring, responsible citizens. The meetings were structured and the boys were expected to participate with respect for the leaders as well as each other. They each played a major role in Trampus's maturing, accepting responsibility, and taking the necessary step toward independence. They not only allowed him to go camping with the troop without us, they encouraged us to let him do so. Up until this time, I had always been involved in helping or just being involved. The one important factor that I have had to continually reinforce with those who work with Trampus: be firm with him and demand his respect for their authority. Although I know that can be very difficult, if they will do this, he can be a joy to work with.

The first camping opportunity came, and fortunately, the campground selected was just down the road from our house. At least if he needed me or if they should need me, I was close by. That was probably the longest Saturday night and Sunday morning of my life. I was constantly tempted to just ride over and peek even though I knew deep down that it was not the thing to do. After listening to me for as long as he could, Vince suggested that I call to see if they could tell me anything. We were assured that he was fine, and believed it would definitely be a mistake to come to the campground.

Finally Sunday morning arrived, and we were able to pick him up (just a little earlier than noted on the sheet). There he was, cleaning up the campsite with all the other scouts. As soon as our eyes met, he came running to me. We grabbed each other and held on, but just for a few minutes. I'm not sure which one of us was fighting the hardest to keep back the tears. What a tremendous hurdle for both of us!

While he was not willing to allow too much conversation concerning his camping venture, and although I knew he missed his "crushed ice and cartoons," I believed it would give him an important "growing up" time that would help produce confidence when I wasn't with him. I think one of the reasons the Troop was so supportive of Trampus and the reason I was confident in turning him over to them was because one of the leaders had informed me from the very first meeting that she had a sister with Down syndrome, and as a result of her exposure, she was bold in making recommendations and taking charge for me. They provided firm but caring demands of Trampus and he responded because he was accustomed to it at home.

Many of our friends knew and understood my desire to encourage others regarding children with special needs so I was not surprised when I was asked to get in touch with a young mother who had just had a little girl with Down syndrome. Trampus was around two years old at the time, and as a result of that phone call, he and I have a very special friendship with two wonderful people—Rebecca and Trista Kutcher. We have been able to share many wonderful times together and have been able to comfort each other when the need arises.

One very important time they were able to be together involved participating in the local Cotillion. My granddaughter had received an invitation and I thought what a perfect place for Trampus and Trista to learn manners and etiquette. This would be one more opportunity to meet others outside of their school and churches. Of course I could hear the concern of the woman that was in charge, but after I pointed out that my understanding of the purpose of the Cotillion was to instruct young men and women on proper behavior in society and I felt this would provide a great opportunity to teach all of them how to do just that as they were sure to meet people in all walks of life. Although I believe she agreed with my logic, I really think they were able to be a part of the group because several of the board members (teacher at Whitesides and a deacon at our church) had opportunities to be with Trampus and Trista and they believed both would be able to participate. They had a wonderful time dressing up and learning the dances. Trampus took immediately to the escorting, door opening, and greetings, while Trista enjoyed guiding him through the dancing. I am convinced it played a very important part in building their confidence and improving their social skills.

Living at the beach, we were an "outdoor" household which always involved boating and sports. One of our "fun" activities was to ride our bikes around the island where we lived. That had been put aside once Trampus was too big to ride in a seat attached to the bike. His dad decided it was time for Trampus to ride a bike so we could return to the island adventure of exploring.

Youch! I still today marvel at the "quitting not an option" attitude of Vince (as is the case in most things that he and/or Trampus desires). The process began. The effort was grueling for all! At one point I remember Ashley and Tripp begging, "Mom, make them stop." Ain't gonna happen. There was a mission to accomplish and that was that. After scraped up knees, elbows, and bike seats, we took one of our "sessions" to the beach. At least there, we would have a softer landing but a firm ground at low tide. What a great idea! Here was the plan: Vince would ride on his bike beside Trampus. I would be the "pusher-offer" and then run alongside for a while.

What a great plan. I did my part. I got him started, ran along beside him until he picked up speed. There he went like a flash; only one problem…his direction. The next few minutes were like slow motion. I was already cold. It was November and we're on the beach, and suddenly Trampus—sweat suit and all—was headed for the ocean. *Yikes!* I can still hear my voice screaming "turn Trampus turn." (Now I think of "run Forest run" in the movie *Forest Gump*.) It reminded me of the quote "riding off into the sunset." The first vision I got as he rode into the surf was the tricycle rider on an old TV series called *Laugh-In*. A large person would ride a tricycle and all of a sudden fall over to the side. When the first wave hit, he just fell over—bike and all—into the water but he kept right on pedaling. Boy, what an experience. The amazing thing was he never quit, so we are able as a family to ride whereever we desire. Go Trampus! I have to admit, though, I think this success came as a desire to please his dad.

Because we had been so committed to raising Trampus in an environment much like that of his sister and brother, and because we felt the importance of peer role modeling, we had not expanded that environment to include the special needs community. When Trampus was young, we received a letter at our business from the Special Olympics South Carolina (SOSC), which is a non-profit organization. They provide a wonderful service for people with special needs, particularly those with Down syndrome. Needless to say, we have a heart for their cause, and while we were not financially able to just write a check toward their work, my husband offered to produce their screen printing services at a much-reduced cost. We have continued to work with them and have grown very close to those involved with the organization.

As we began to meet the screen printing and embroidery needs for SOSC, we took the opportunity to deliver the shirts in person to one of the summer games so that we could see firsthand what was being accomplished. We felt this would be a great opportunity to introduce Trampus to people who experienced some of the same difficulties. The games were being played in the same town where we had family, so we would deliver the shirts and then go back and get Trampus for the opening ceremonies. What happened next was a total surprise! Trampus began to look around, and within a short amount of time, made it very clear that he was uncomfortable and wanted to leave and go back to his grandmother's. He was looking at the special needs participants in the very same way I had seen people look at him. Once again I could see God guiding us into an opportunity to help him learn how to interact with all people. We wanted him to learn the very thing he had taught us. I never realized until then that we would need to teach him how to include others just as we had asked others to include him.

I knew it wasn't that he was thoughtless or mean, it was just exactly what I had experienced, and many like us; we just don't know how to be a part of an environment that is unfamiliar. Through our involvement with SOSC, we have been able to expose him and allow him to learn how very special each person is; how each person deserves his kindness and respect. His natural gift is being thoughtful and encouraging to those around him, but we had to encourage him not to be selective with his gift. Rather, he needed to give it freely since it had been given freely to him.

When we returned from that weekend, I knew we needed to get involved in some form of unified activities. Once again, a door opened that allowed us to participate in a soccer league that had been started as a buddy league. Each special needs child had a peer that played by his/her side. The intention was for the buddy to provide as little or as much help as needed.

While Trampus needed little help other than learning the skills, it allowed him to watch children helping children and taught him that although some children weren't able to participate at the same level, they were still able to be a part of the team. As they all began to cheer for each other and became familiar with each other, walls of separation began to fall. Soon they were a team and totally unaware of any differences, proving once again that it is not the differences that alienate us, but the fear and lack of understanding regarding those differences.

We decided to expose Trampus to the world of gymnastics through Tapio School of Dance and Gymnastics. This is where his friend Trista trained. Susan Breland is incredible in working with all children regardless of their abilities. Through the training Trista received, she has successfully competed with fellow students, and has won gold medals in the Special Olympics South Carolina competitions including the World Games in Ireland. Trampus enjoyed his time with Susan and I believe it provided him the opportunity to build strength not only in his legs and arms, but his total person. In addition to the strength training, he was required to learn the routines which helped his sequencing skills. I regret we didn't get seriously involved when he was younger because, although he enjoyed it, his love for sports and music won over the time and effort required to continue in gymnastics.

The local recreation department offered a unified sports league and for a while Trampus enjoyed participating in the various sports. What fun to watch his excitement when he would hear the screams and applause when he would "make a basket" or "make a goal." While it was a fun time for him, as he grew and the demands grew with his music, we had to pull away. I wish he could have done both so that his relationships with the "special needs" community could have grown deeper also.

These are the experiences that many desire, but few experience. We are very thankful for a community that has been so compassionate and supportive.

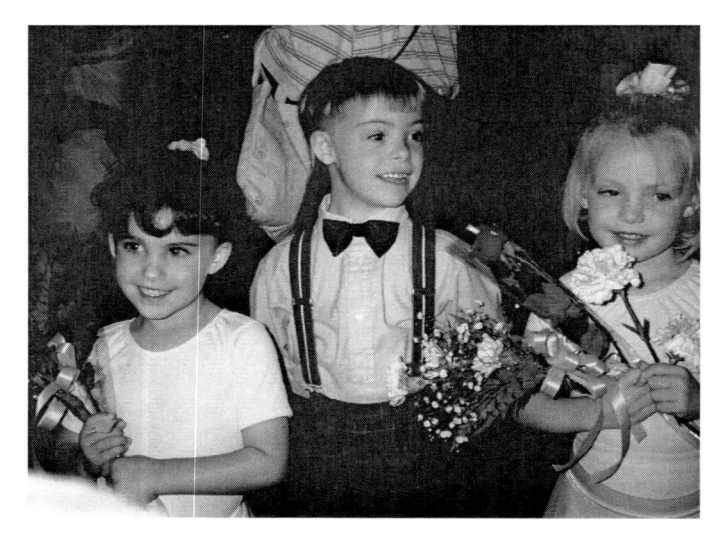

Trampus with niece Emily and her cousin Morgan

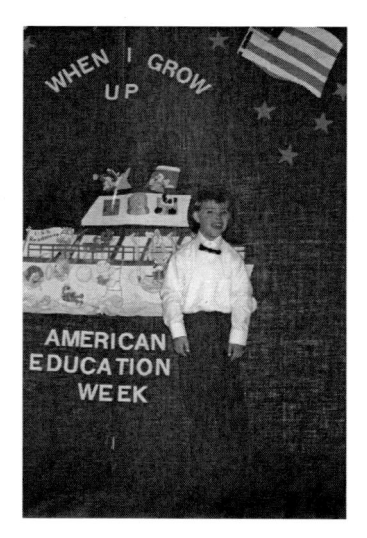

Whiteside's Elementary performance

Down Strong

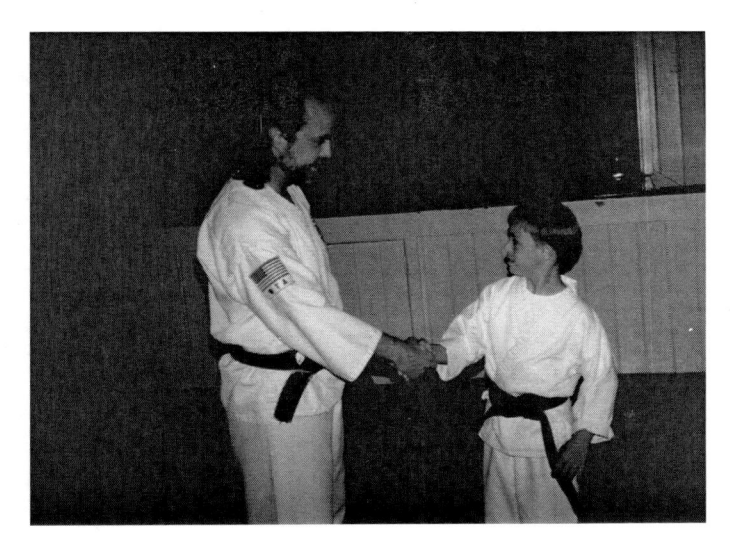

Receiving Green Belt in karate

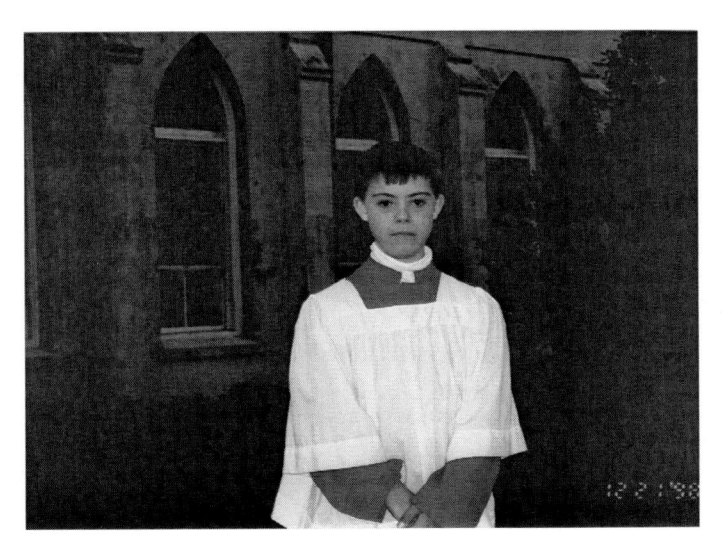

Altar Server

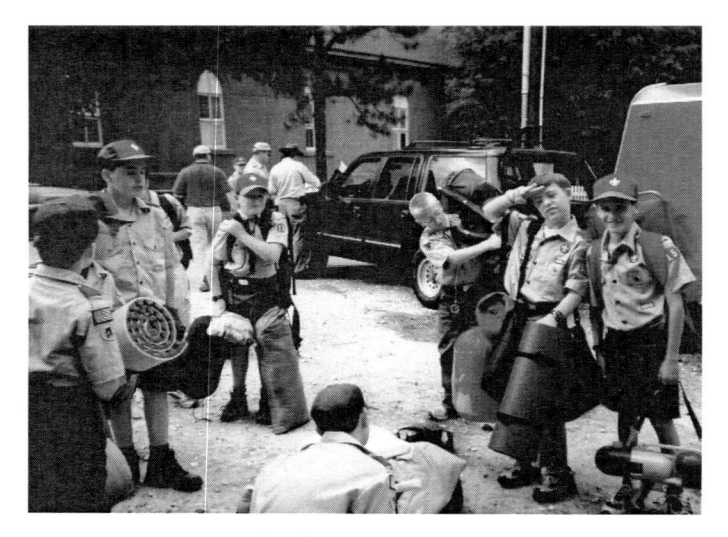

Boy Scout camping trip

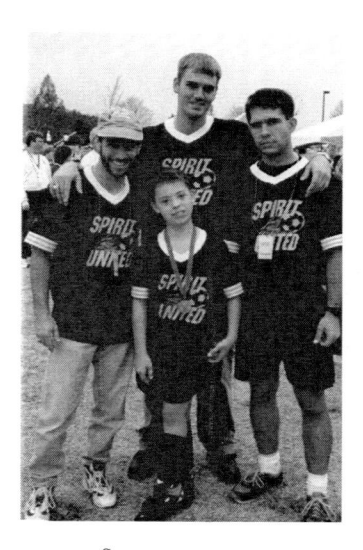

Soccer tournament

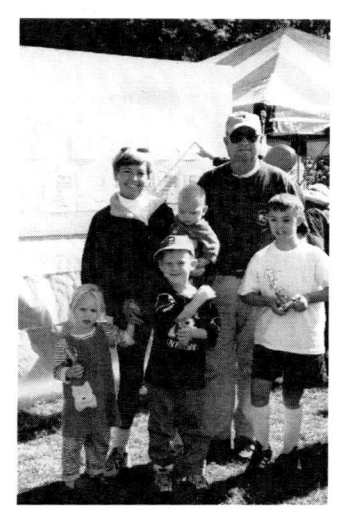

Mom, Dad and grandchildren Vincent, Daniel, Elizabeth with Trampus at tournament

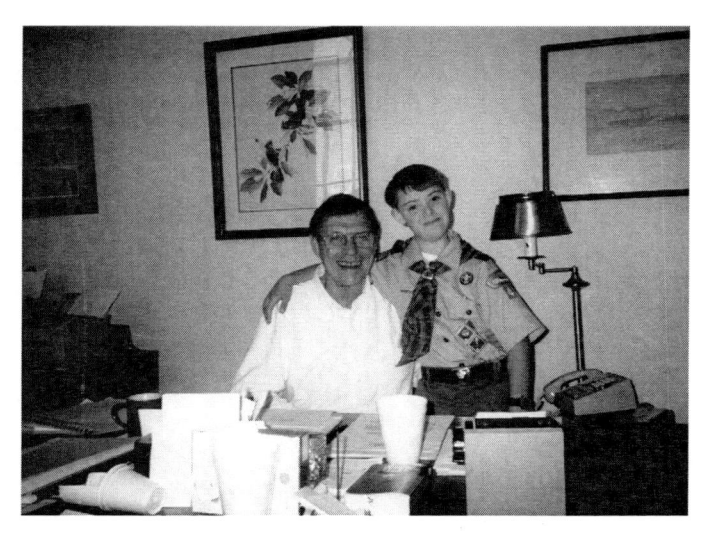

Trampus and Senator Arthur Ravenel

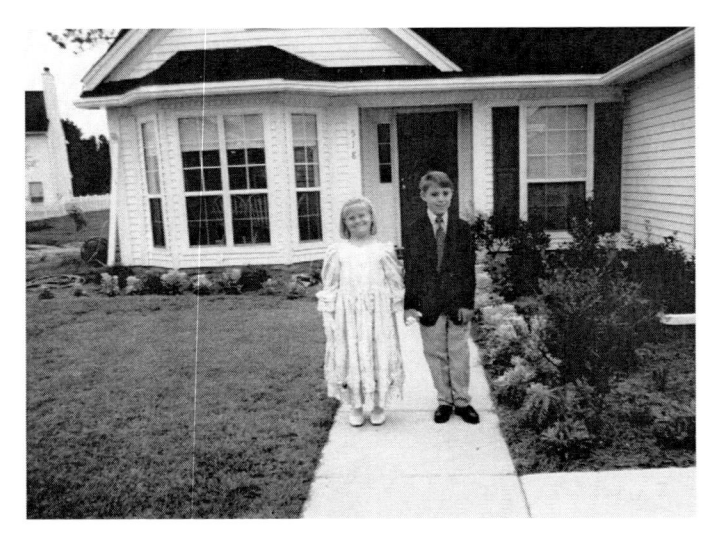

Trampus and Trista headed to their first Cotillion

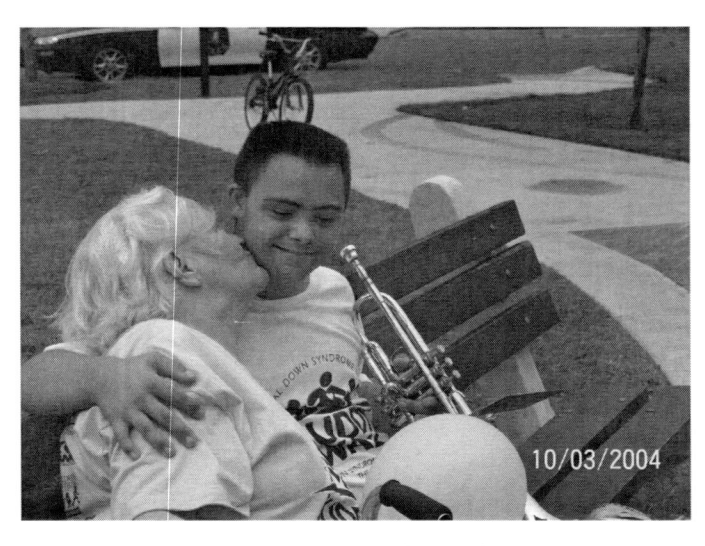

*Trampus getting a kiss from Trista's "Grammy"—
played Amazing grace at her funeral*

Down Strong

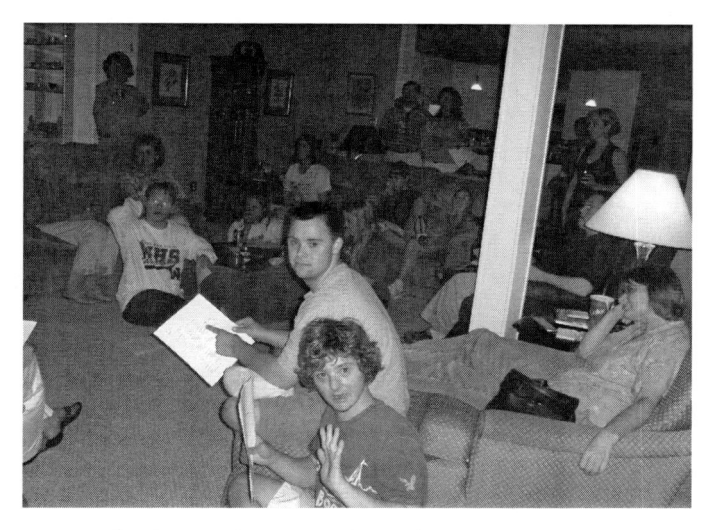

Co-chairman Trampus at Down Syndrome Association of the Lowcountry Advocate Youth Group meeting

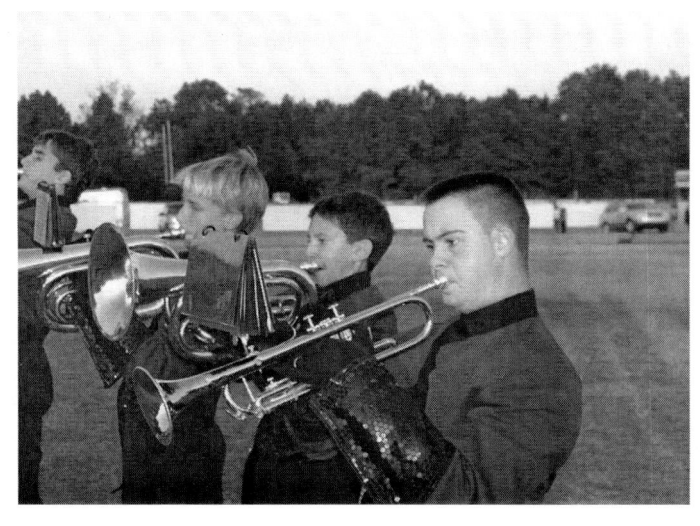

Warming up for Wando football game half-time performance

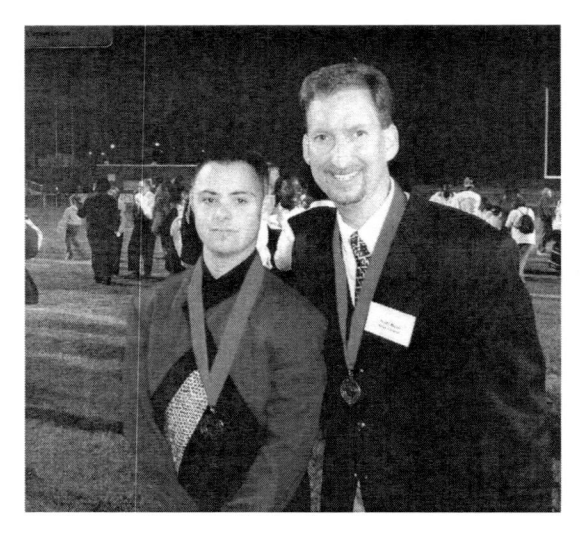

Trampus with Wando High School Band Director, Scott Rush, after receiving his SC State 5A Marching Band Championship medal

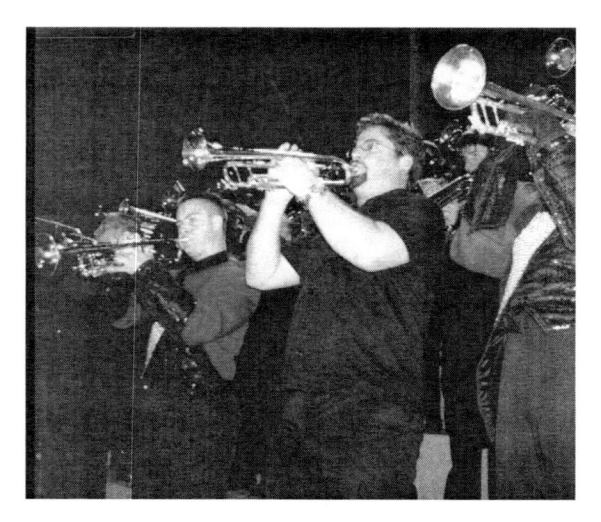

Trampus and Laing Band Director, Jeremy Rohr, jamming in stands at football game

Down Strong

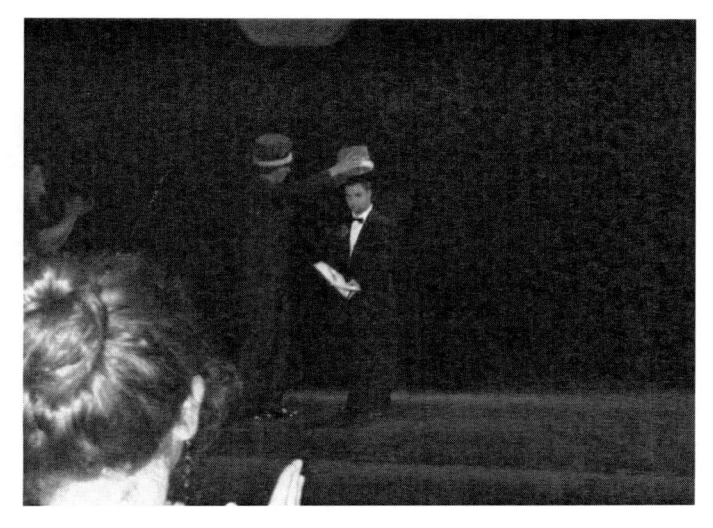

Receiving crown after being named Mr. Wando

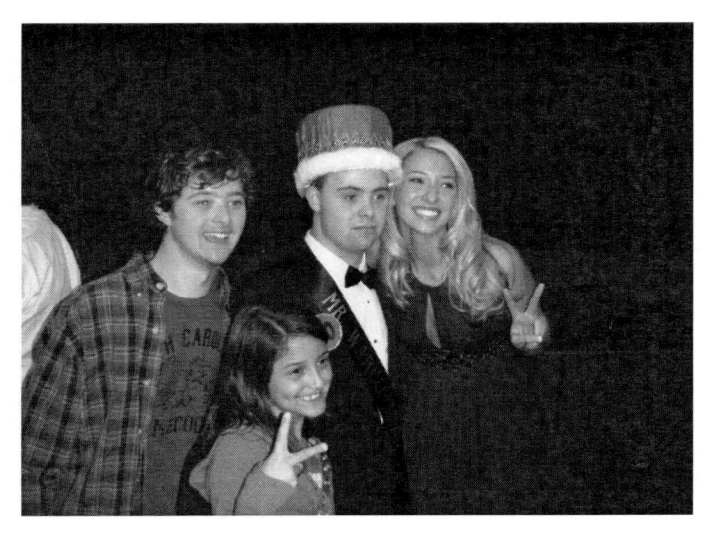

Trampus with his escort Jessie Gravino, her sister Lexi, and brother Zach

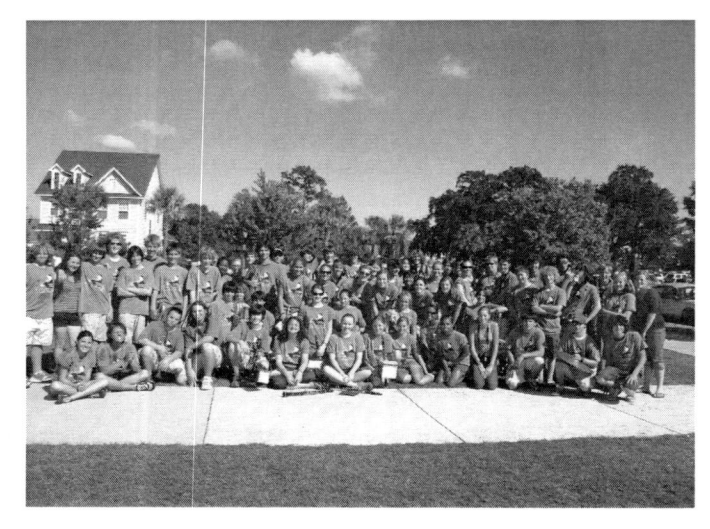

Wando Band with Trampus at the DSAL Buddy Walk

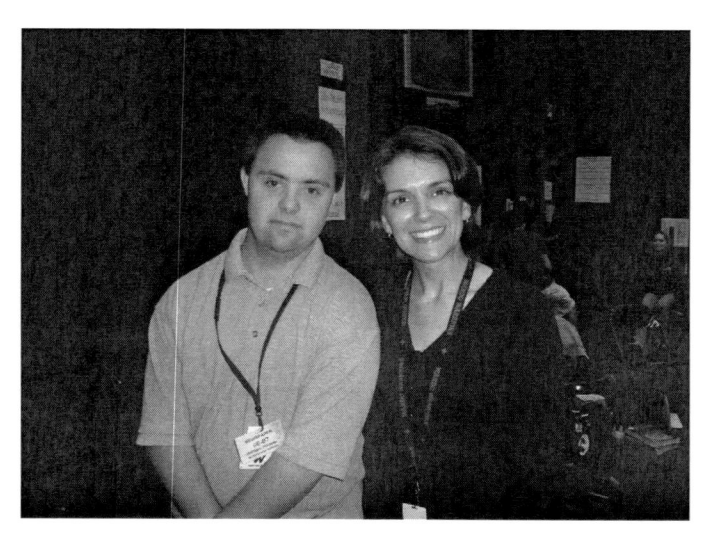

Trampus with Drama teacher, Selina May

Down Strong

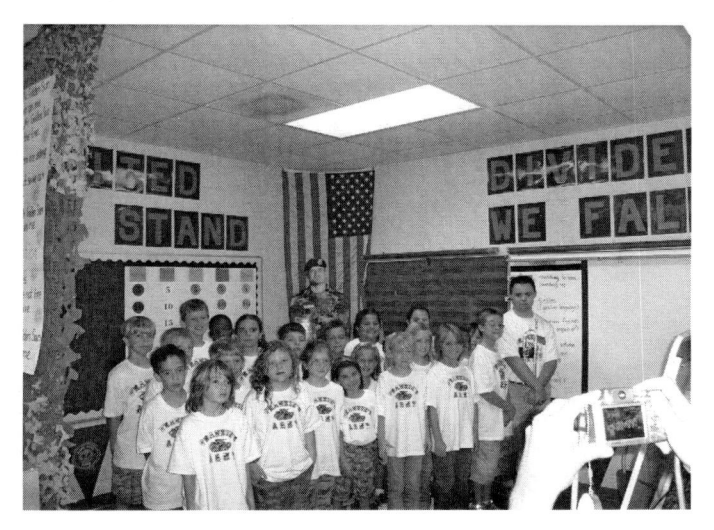

Trampus at Pinckney Elementary School giving a speech on advocacy and playing a few Disney tunes on his trumpet for the class

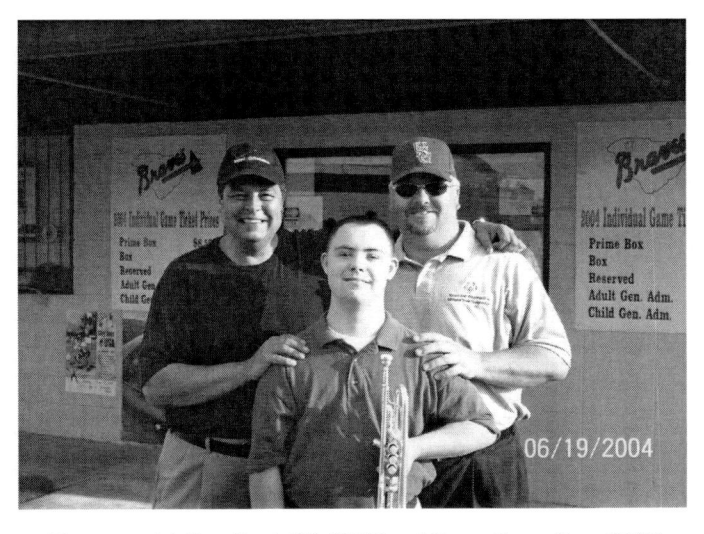

Trampus with Ray Carci, VP, SOSC and Barry Coats, Pres, SOSC before playing National Anthem at Greenville Braves baseball game

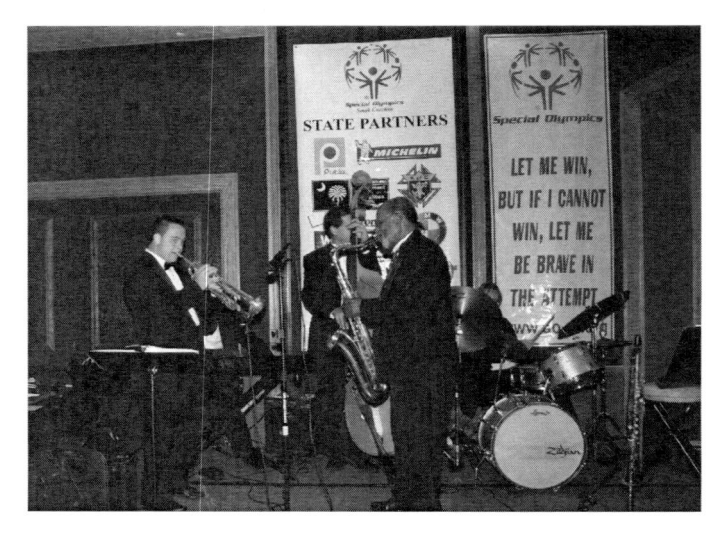

Trampus playing with Skipp Pearson, member of the SC Jazz Hall of Fame at the SOSC Gala in Columbia, SC

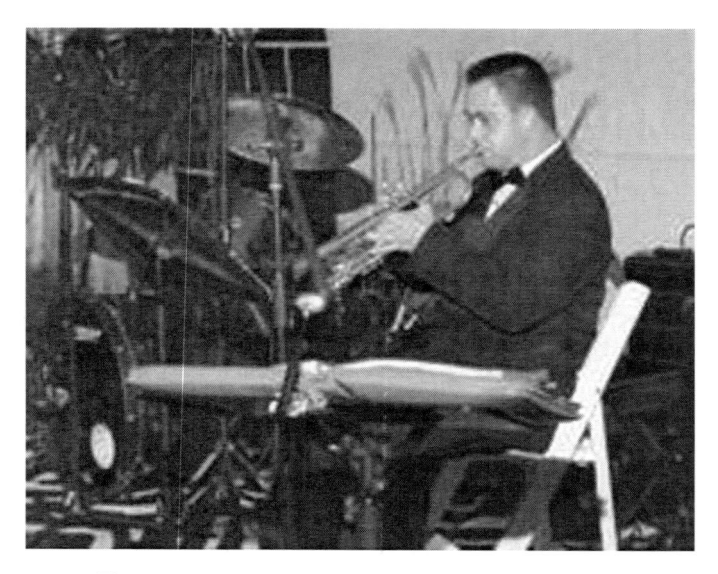

Trampus performing at the SOSC Gala in Charleston, SC

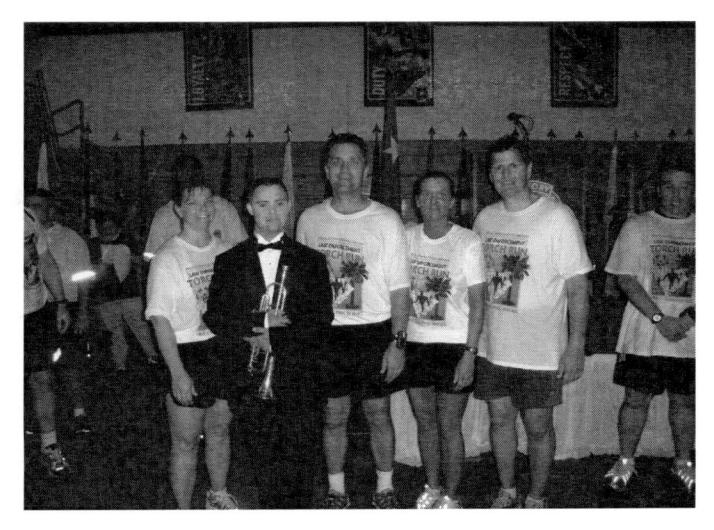

Trampus played National Anthem for summer games after the SC Law Enforcement Officers brought torch in for SOSC Summer Games

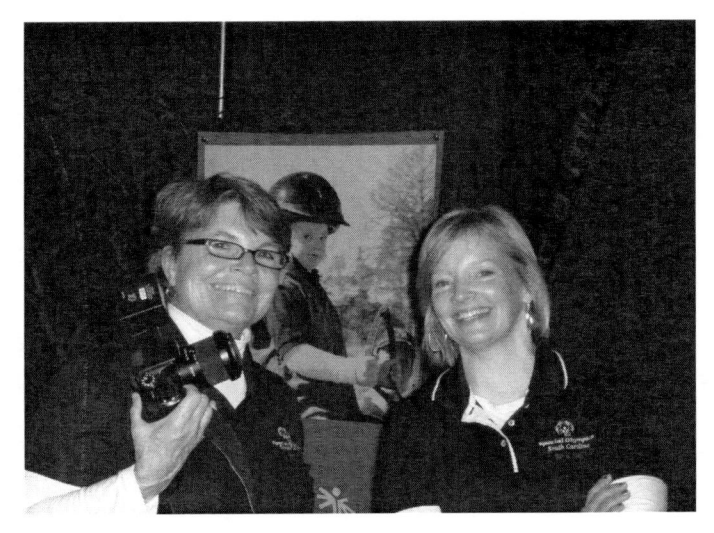

Sue Maner, Exec VP, SOSC and Kelly Garrick, Director of Sports, coordinating Mid-winter Games

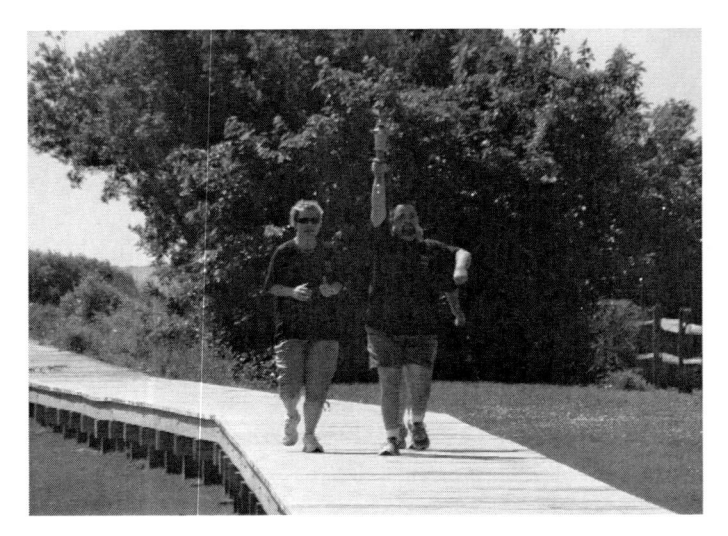

*Trampus beginning the Coast to Capital Run
for the SOSC Summer Games*

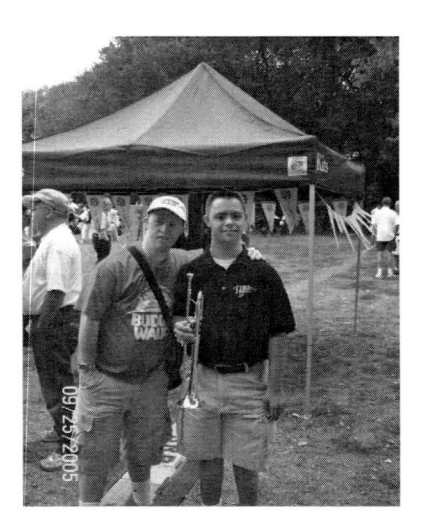

*Trampus with Chris Burke, star of series "Life Goes On"
in Central Park at the New York Buddy Walk where
Trampus opened by playing the National Anthem*

Down Strong

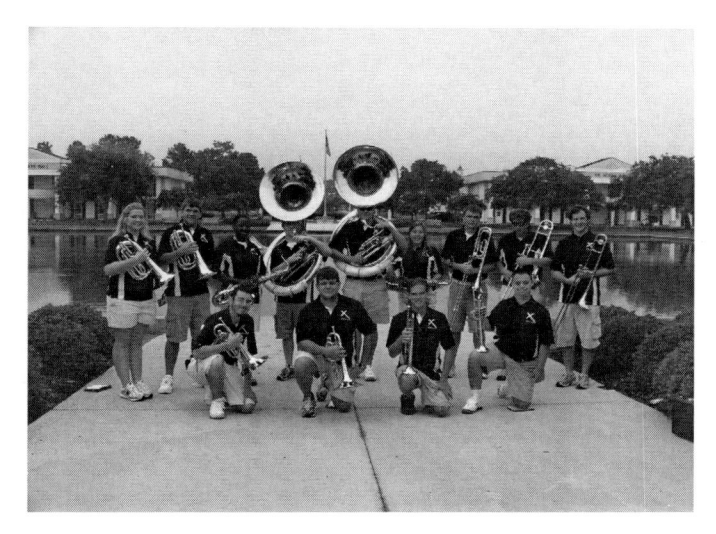

Brass band at Charleston Southern University

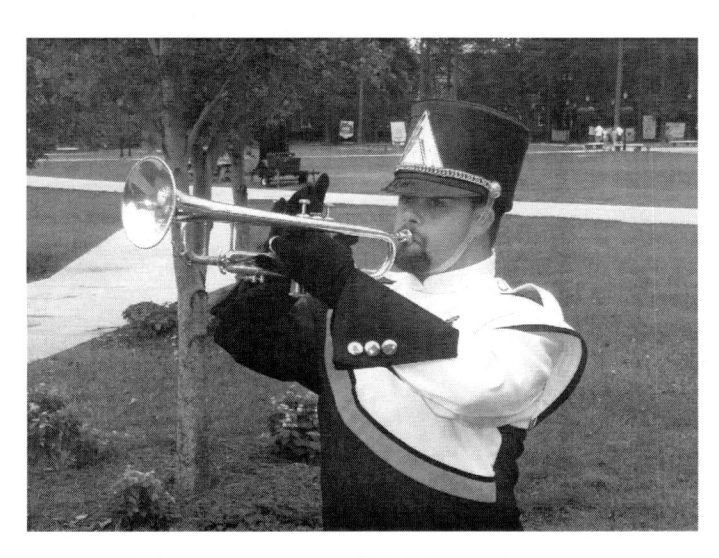

Trampus warming up for half-time performance at Coastal Carolina University

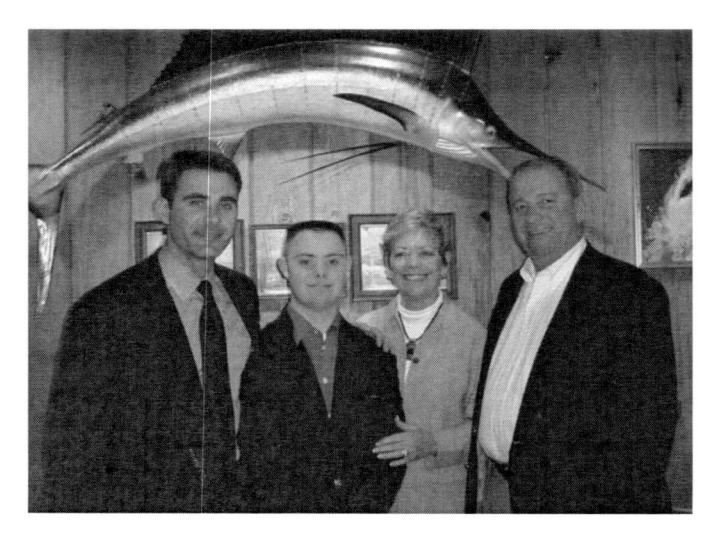

Trampus, Mom, Dad and Lt. Gov Andre Bauer

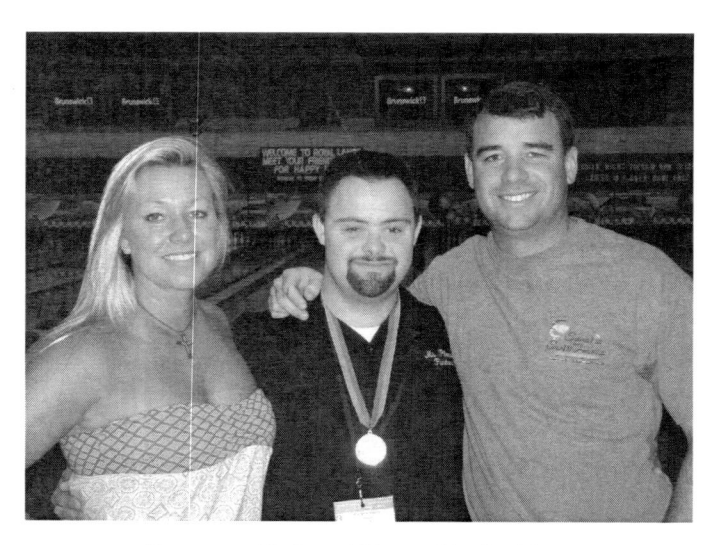

Trampus with sister Ashley, and brother Tripp, at SOSC Bowling Tournament

Down Strong

Elizabeth, Ashley, Tripp, Eliza, Mom, Andrew, Vincent Manning and Trampus at SOSC Bowling Tournament

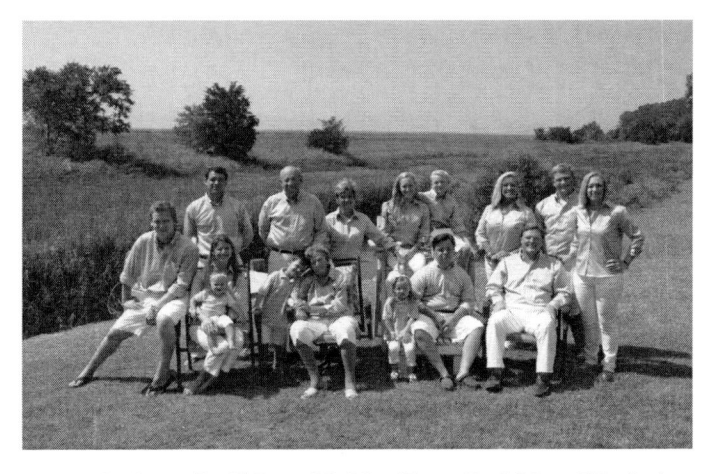

Family photo: (Back) Daniel Bolchoz, Tripp, Dad, Mom, Elizabeth Bolchoz, Manning Bolchoz, Ashley Bolchoz, Vincent Bolchoz, Emily Bolchoz (Front) Kristy Hoover, Caroline Hoover, Andrew Hoover, Louise Hoover (Gommy), Eliza Hoover, Trampus, Mark Bolchoz

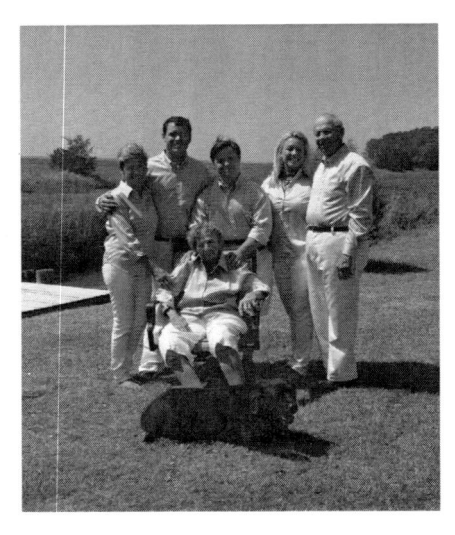

Mom, Tripp, Trampus, Ashley, Dad, Gommy and dog Buddy

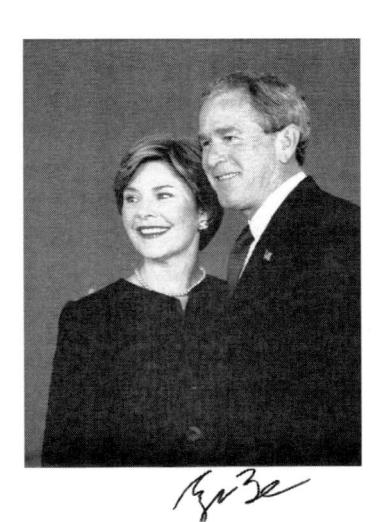

Autographed picture of President George W. Bush and Laura Bush

Down Strong

THE WHITE HOUSE
WASHINGTON

April 4, 2007

Trampus Hoover
1520 Lieben Road
Mount Pleasant, South Carolina 29466-9134

Dear Trampus:

I recently learned some wonderful things about you.

Young Americans can make a difference in our country by studying hard, making right choices, and helping others. I hope you will continue to set high goals and strive to learn something new every day. Your idealism and energy reflect the spirit of our Nation.

Mrs. Bush and I send our best wishes.

Sincerely,

George W. Bush

Letter of congratulations from the President of the United States, George W. Bush for receiving the "International Yes I Can Award".

Martha Stewart Hoover

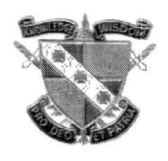

Hanahan High School

6015 MURRAY AVENUE · HANAHAN, SOUTH CAROLINA 29410
PHONE (843) 820-3710 · FAX (843) 820-3716

Dr. Glenda LeVine
Principal

May 2, 2009

To Whom it May Concern,

    I am writing this letter of recommendation on behalf of Trampus Hoover. I have had the pleasure of knowing Trampus for the past nine years. I have worked with him in the capacity of his private trumpet instructor, and as an instructor with the Wando High School marching band. I have been lucky to be a part of this amazing young man's life. I still do not know who learned more, he or I, from our time together.

    In the time I have know Trampus, I have watched him grow into a true musician. Trampus has an immense joy for life, which becomes very evident when he plays his trumpet. The pride he takes in playing for other people is very inspiring to watch. His ability to master the higher-level skills needed to play the trumpet has continued to amaze me. Trampus had one goal when working with me, and that was to learn to play the trumpet. The focus and drive he developed while working towards that goal, put him on par, if not ahead, of his peers in band.

    Through his dedication and determination, Trampus has earned a chair in many ensembles and honor clinics. Some of the ensembles he has auditioned for and earned a place in, being: Wando High School's concert band, Wando High School's marching Band, The University of South Carolina Band Clinic, Charleston County All-County Honor Clinic, South Carolina Band Director's Region IV Honor Clinic, and Charleston Southern University's marching band. His accomplishments have not come without hard work and frustrations, but no musicians' accomplishments come without lots of "blood, sweat, and tears."

    I have seen Trampus achieve amazing things. He has accomplished things no one ever thought he would be able to do. But Trampus is a diligent and strong-minded individual, who wants to learn all he can about the things he is passionate for. I truly believe Trampus is very deserving of your scholarship, and will be nothing but successful at the endeavors this opportunity will open up for him.

Sincerely,

Dr. Gretchen Bowles
Band Director/String Specialist
Hanahan High School
843-820-3710 ext 2001

Letter of recommendation for the "International Yes I Can Award" from Dr. Gretchen Bowles, Band Director, Hanahan High School

Down Strong

Town of Mount Pleasant

Harry M. Hallman, Jr.
Mayor

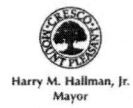

May 20, 2009

To Whom This May Concern:

Trampus Hoover has been an inspirational citizen to the Town of Mount Pleasant. When asked, he has always accepted any request to play his trumpet for Town events. This very talented young man has played for athletic events that the Town has sponsored, bringing in visitors from many states, and has kicked off the gymnastics competition for Special Olympics South Carolina held in Mount Pleasant. He has served in this capacity not only for his Town, but throughout the state as well.

Trampus has also honored our fallen officers who have given their lives while serving the tri-county area. As a result of his hard work and commitment to the Town of Mount Pleasant, Mayor Harry M. Hallman, Jr. awarded him the key to the Town in 2005. We are very fortunate that such a dedicated, amazing young man calls the Town of Mount Pleasant home.

Sincerely yours,

Kruger B. Smith
Mayor Pro Tem
TOWN OF MOUNT PLEASANT

KBS:cb

P.O. Box 745 • 100 Ann Edwards Lane • Mount Pleasant, SC 29465 • (843) 884-8517 • Fax (843) 856-218

Letter of recommendation from the Pro-Tem Mayor of Mt Pleasant, SC, Kruger Smith for the "International Yes I Can Award."

INSPIRE GREATNESS

Special Olympics
South Carolina

Officers
Teri Buonasera, Chair
 Chernoff, Newman
James Price, Vice Chair
 Price, Pascal, &
 Ashmore
John Moore, Treasurer
 JMI Consultants
Shelly Clark, Secretary
 Wachovia
Michael Mueller
 Palmetto Elder Law
John Tully
 Michelin North America
Frank Antonelli
 Empire Sports
Tom Gilligan
 Colonial Supplemental

Directors
Terry Ansley
 Colliers Keenan, LLC
John Bradford
 Athlete Representative
Howard Buonasera
 Cablevantage
Bennie Cunningham
 Retired NFL – Steelers
Andy DeMasi
 Carolina First
Sharon Gulshy
 Michelin
Jane Hughes-Warner
 City of Spartanburg
Sheriff Leon Lott
 Richland County
 Sheriff's Department
Larry Lucas
 State Farm
Susan Luttman
 Dept. of Mental Health
Suzanne McMahan
 Anderson County
 Special Populations
Matthew Miller
 Northwest Mutual
Diana Poiletman
 Athlete Representative
Richard Stachelek
 Knights of Columbus

President & CEO
Barry S. Coats

To Whom It May Concern:

Picture 1,000 Special Olympics athletes and coaches, 2,000 soldiers and 250 family members packed into Fort Jackson's Solomon Center. Then picture Trampus Hoover standing on stage playing the National Anthem on his trumpet. Now try to picture a dry eye!

During a Special Olympics event at the Citadel, Trampus impressed the college sports staff so much that they invited him to play at the opening of their basketball conference playoffs. He has played at many local, state, and even national events – not because he has Down syndrome, but because he is good! Trampus even played the National Anthem at Times Square last year to kick off the New York City Buddy Walk.

Trampus made Wando High School's band (AAAAA State Champions) by auditioning behind a curtain so the panel only heard his musical ability. His band members now are his biggest supporters when he competes in Special Olympics. He brought a third of the band to the local Buddy Walk in Charleston and now they are all backing him for the Polar Plunge fundraiser to be held in January.

Trampus' greatest talent though, may be his easy way of fitting into his community. People at his school and community look as his abilities and not his disabilities when they meet Trampus and spend time with him.

On top of being the President of Special Olympics, I am also the proud parent of a seven-year old daughter, Erin, with Down syndrome. Even in the world I work in, there are still many unknowns for what I can expect for Erin. Without knowing it, Trampus gives me the greatest gift that I could ever ask for – hope. When I see what Trampus has accomplished I know Erin doesn't have to be held back by what some would call a disability. She can set goals and work to accomplish them.

If I can be of any further assistance please call me at 803-772-1555 ext.313 or email at Bcoats@so-sc.org.

Regards,

Barry S. Coats
President & CEO

810 Dutch Square Blvd. Suite 204 / Columbia, SC 29210
P.O. Box 210099 / Columbia, SC 29221-0099
Phone: 803.772.1555 / Fax: 803.772.0094 / Website: www.SO-SC.org

Letter of recommendation for the "International Yes I Can Award" from Barry Coats, President, Special Olympics South Carolina

Down Strong

WANDO HIGH SCHOOL BAND

November 15, 2006

Recommendation: Trampus Hoover

To Whom It May Concern:

I am writing this letter of recommendation on behalf of Trampus Hoover, a student in the Wando High School Band program. I have had the privilege of teaching Trampus for the past four years and feel that I am uniquely qualified to give this assessment.

Trampus is a remarkable person who has gone *above and beyond* in the world of music. Logic would dictate that a young man with Down's syndrome would not be able to function in a nationally recognized band program. However, Trampus defies the odds. He doesn't possess a special gift toward music, he simply works harder than anyone else. What he does possess is a passion and love for music-making! Because of this fact, he is an incredible role model for students within our program. Trampus has improved tremendously and has progressed each year in our chair placement auditions. He plays his trumpet for local and national functions and is a wonderful ambassador for the Wando community.

It is my belief that Trampus will continue to positively affect people after high school. If Trampus can share the gift of music with other Down's syndrome kids, it would allow him to thrive in an area in which he is so passionate.

Trampus receives my highest recommendation.

Sincerely,

Scott B. Rush
Director of Bands
(843) 856-2352

1000 WARRIOR WAY • MT. PLEASANT, SC • 29466
PHONE: (843) 881-8257 • FAX: (843) 375-3536

Letter of recommendation for the "International Yes I Can Award" from Scott Rush, Band Director, Wando High School

Martha Stewart Hoover

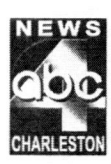

WCIV
ABC News 4

PO Box 22165
Charleston, SC
29413-2165

843.881.4444
www.abcnews4.com

I'VE OFTEN HEARD THAT "LIFE IS 10% WHAT HAPPENS TO YOU AND 90% HOW YOU RESPOND TO IT."

IF THIS IS TRUE THEN TRAMPUS HOOVER IN JUST 18 SHORT YEARS HAS MASTERED THE ART OF LIFE.

TRAMPUS MAY HAVE BEEN BORN SHORT OF A CHROMOSOME BUT HE IS A LIVING EXAMPLE OF SOMEONE WHO'S NEVER BEEN CHEATED OUT OF A DAY.

FROM HIS INFECTIOUS SMILE, TO HIS MAGNANIAMOUS ATTITUDE TRAMPUS IS A SOURCE OF HAPPINESS AND INSPIRATION TO THOSE WHO COME INTO CONTACT WITH HIM.

HIS DEDICATION AND DESIRE TO BE THE VERY BEST IN HIS MUSICAL PURSUIT HAVE LEFT AUDIENCES ASKING FOR MORE. I KNOW THIS FOR FACT BECAUSE I'VE SEEN HIM PLAY FIRST HAND. I'VE HEARD THE AUDIENCE RESPONSE AND I'VE SEEN THE SMILES STRETCH FOR MILES. .

I'VE SPENT TIME WITH THE YOUNG TRUMPETEER WHILE PROFILING HIM FOR OUR LOCAL NEWS BROADCAST. HE IS DESERVING OF ALL THAT COMES HIS WAY AND I CONSIDER HIM TO BE A CHAMPION IN OUR COMMUNITY AS SOMEONE WHO MAKES A DIFFERENCE.

DEAN STEPHENS
ABC NEWS 4
6, 7, AND 11 PM ANCHOR

WCIV, LLC, an Allbritton Group Station

Letter of recommendation for the "International Yes I Can Award" from Dean Stephens, Anchor for ABC News Mt Pleasant, SC

Down Strong

NOTES

8:30 pm Dinner on The Seine

THURSDAY Night w/ M. HOOVER & BILLY SUNDAY

I LOVE You

17 Oct 85

PARIS

Harpist played "what child is This" Next to us at 9:00 pm

THE BARBIZON
Lexington Avenue at 63rd Street, NY
Direct Restaurant Reservations
(212) 715-6929

MIDDLE SCHOOL

Throughout elementary school, Trampus enjoyed an active life of inclusion. He was able to be a part of what was going on with little to no notice of difference. The wonderful thing was that even if there were noticeable differences, the children didn't care. I knew, however, as we moved to the next level of school life, it could prove more difficult. Again, I chose not to play it out in my mind. I would not allow myself to imagine struggles or negative possibilities that could lay in front of us, but met each day with excitement and anticipation. I kept with the mindset that had brought me this far, to trust the desires I would begin to have for Trampus. I anticipated doors would open that would lead us to success. I reminded myself that he was created for a purpose, as is every life, and we would continue to move forward with our goals.

Our friends, Rebecca and Joe Kutcher, whom I mentioned earlier, both taught at Laing Middle School and continuously encouraged us to come and visit the school prior to enrolling. They believed it was important to give Trampus an opportunity to become familiar with the surroundings before becoming a part of it. Because there was no school the day we visited, we were able to meet the librarian and talk with her one on one. Trampus and Ms. Swindle became friends immediately. Her love for children and for her work permeated her very being. She had a morning TV announcement channel that would play into each classroom and so she let Trampus talk and see himself on the TV screen. Being the performer that he is, he accepted her offer of being a part of the *WLNG* "gang" with excitement. He now began to let go of his hold on Whitesides Elementary and began to look forward to becoming a Laing Middle School student. Of course, our successful life at Laing would never have been possible without the support of the administration and faculty. Principal Dr. Kathy Sobolewski, and Assistant Principal Ms. Deborah Price (Trampus referred to her as "Ms. Priceless"). They were not only open to recommendations offered by the school community, they were creative and active in making some of their own. What a great example of how community effort will produce success!

I knew that the possibility of Trampus continuing in the regular classroom would become more and more difficult. Each class would require its own demand and the speed in which the learning took place would multiply tremendously.

Our resource connection at Laing was Jan Holzberger. Jan and Rebecca worked closely together to help the "middle school" world open up to new ways of inclusion. I have to include a funny story about Jan and Trampus. In our discussions with what we felt was best for Trampus, Jan had made it very clear that she felt he should be made aware of the fact that he had

Down syndrome. Vince and I had decided early on that unless he asked or gave some inclination of interest, we would continue to discuss the fact that he was better at some things, and required more help in others with no explanation as to why. One day when I came to pick Trampus up, Jan pulled me off to the side. She said, "I give up. I determined today that Trampus is not interested in any type of categorization." She went on to say that while she had several of the children with Down syndrome in a room together for resource, she decided to use a teaching moment. She pointed out to each of them that most people with Down syndrome have a straight line that ran across the palms of their hands. She watched each one look down into their palms. As she watched each child's reaction, heads moving up and down acknowledging the lines, she came to Trampus and their eyes met. He looked down at his palm, closed it quickly, and very matter-of-factly looked up at her and said "nope." It was interesting; however, that not too long after that, we were eating breakfast in a restaurant and a mother with a young child on her hip came up to our table. She asked if I was Martha Hoover and when I acknowledged that I was, she went on to say that she also had a son with Down syndrome and inquired if it was okay to meet to talk about Trampus. "Awkward." When we exchanged phone numbers and she walked away, Vince and I looked at each other and waited on a comment from Trampus… nothing. That night when Trampus and I were saying his prayers, he asked me, "Mom, why do people know me?" I was able to take that time and explain: "Trampus, when you were born, we were told by the doctors that you had an 'extra chromosome' and that because of it, life could be very difficult for you. Other babies are born with that same extra chromosome and other parents hear the same thing. The 'so-called' problem is Down syndrome. It can make moms and dads very sad to think their children may have a hard time so when people see you and see all that you can do and have accomplished, it makes them happy. It helps take away the fear they may feel for their child. They want their babies to be able to have a chance to do all the things you are able to do." What a special moment for the two of us; definitely a "God timing" thing. He looked up at me, smiled, and said "oh!" That night began the acceptance and acknowledgement of Down syndrome in the life of William Sunday Trampus Hoover. This was confirmation for us, of our decision to allow him to choose the time.

Although there were and still are times when I admit I experience concern and confusion about direction and purpose, if I resolve not to become anxious and back off from the situation allowing time, it will always result in what's best not only for Trampus, but others that are involved. The greatest gift we can give our children concerning their education, as well as general life skills while under our care, is to be a part of it, but doing so as part of the solution, not the problem. Our fear can trigger an unnecessary defense mechanism unless we guard our emotions. Our reaction can produce success or encourage failure. The success will come when everyone stays concerned about all involved;

not each taking a stand for self regardless of what it cost the other. Someone has to take the first step and I have found if I make that effort, then everyone seems to follow.

With the cooperation of all the people involved with Trampus, whether faculty, staff, friends, or just acquaintants, Trampus continues to shine and carry the light of hope for those who must work harder at not only finding their gift, but also using it in the community around them.

We decided within a short time that Trampus would not flourish in the regular education program, so we agreed for him to become a part of the Educable Mental Disabled (EMD) self-contained classroom. The teacher, Nadine Gomez, helped Trampus realize his potential and provided an environment that bred success. She designed a curriculum that tied in with the regular education program but was adapted to the necessary level of learning. The schedule was the same each day so that once the children learned that, they were able to concentrate on the information being presented. This proved to be tremendously important for Trampus because it gave him the ability to give full focus to the subject matter which allowed him to succeed. By enjoying good grades, he was willing to continue to put forth the effort.

The need for a self-contained classroom might have been disturbing had there not been opportunity for inclusion in other school-oriented activities. Of course, he would have homeroom and his elective subjects, along with *WLNG*, but our hope was to provide an environment that involved social interaction with all of the students. Rebecca Kutcher had decided to start an exclusive "by invitation only" club. Peers would be selected who would offer good role modeling, showed interest in helping, and who had an overall compassion for people with different needs. Trampus was invited to participate as one of the charter members. As the program began to unfold, Rebecca found out about a grant program initiated by Dr. Conway Saylor called "Peer Express." Although Dr. Conway does not have a child with special needs, she continuously champions the way for our children by proving the positive effect they have not only in education, but in the community. In no time, the program was an incredible success and expanded to include the other two middle schools east of the Cooper. This provided an opportunity for our children to have a social life outside of academics. This program not only brought the children together, but also drew the families together which created a close community spirit. Many times the new families would come into the performances very serious and stiff. In no time, faces were smiling, hands were clapping, and the whole place would be rocking. What fun to share our children with others and to see their differences and similarities enjoyed by all! How blessed we are to have people like Dr. Saylor, who have the kind of insight and determination to find ways to open doors and make inclusion possible for all that desire it! The most amazing thing about this beautiful lady and her family is that they give without having a need. Her husband

and children were not only willing to give her up to be with us, they would give of their time and talent as well.

I love the story of Trampus's involvement with the Laing Middle School Band. Although Trampus had enjoyed his music at the elementary level, I knew it would be difficult to pursue it through chorus. Singing was definitely not his strength and the competition would only get more intense as he got older. One area that started to come to my mind was the band. Surely he could play something like the drums or cymbals, or maybe just be in the band and help keep up with the instruments. I wanted him to be involved with something I knew he loved. He has a wonderful sense of rhythm, so I was convinced that if the director would give him a chance, he could play a positive and helpful role in the band.

I had expressed my desire and intentions to pursue band with several people, but most felt it would be a mistake. Sequencing is very difficult, so their belief was I would be putting him in a situation that would be too difficult which would set him up for failure. Thank goodness the vision I had inside was greater than what I was receiving from the outside. This is another example of the need to keep moving forward with a desire even if it seems impossible. We must remember that many of our successes are enjoyed as a result of stepping out in faith rather than accepting the expectations or lack of expectations of those around us.

I think the real miracle in Trampus's participation in the Laing Middle School Band was the fact that I decided to read the Laing newsletter a particular morning in July, although it had actually been received in May. The intention of the letter was to provide information for new students entering the school. As I read through the information, I realized that day was the very last day for students to come by and talk with the band director and get tested for an instrument. I have always felt strongly that if we want the same opportunity as others, we must, where possible, do what others had to do. Therefore, we could not miss this day to request a place in the band.

Before I had time to even think, I was dressed, Trampus was showered, and we were on our way to Laing Middle School. The band director, Ms. Christina Schneider (now Doctor), was in the office when we arrived. After a short conversation she told me that she had heard of our interest (I'm sure through the Kutchers). She invited us to follow her to the band room so that she could test and see if there was a place for him in the band. I remember thinking, *Oh gosh, I was just hoping she was going to let him help her out with equipment, or handing out papers, and here she is testing him…ugh! Oh well, we'll keep moving forward until the door closes.*

I waited outside the door. I like to think it was so that I would not distract Trampus, but in reality I think I was too nervous to watch. After their session together, she was quick to point out that she didn't have a need for student helpers because the parents handled that. However, she was willing to give him an opportunity to learn the trumpet. As much as I had believed this was what we wanted, I could hardly believe my ears.

Suddenly, I thought this time I just might have gotten myself in over my head. She explained her decision. Trampus had a music language; therefore, she believed there was a good chance he could learn the trumpet. We asked Trampus if this was what he wanted and there was no hesitation; he wanted to begin right then. She was so encouraging and seemed so confident, I made up my mind that because Trampus wanted this and she was willing to work with him and find a tutor, we were going to be successful.

Trampus and I left that meeting, went home, and I researched trumpets. By the time Vince arrived home from work, I had determined which trumpet we wanted and that we purchase it and not rent it. Many students rent before committing. To rent it would say we could quit. No way! Trampus was going to need this instrument forever!

Before I knew it, school had started and our band experience had begun. Although I had the advantage of reading music and playing the piano, I knew nothing about the trumpet. Christy expressed her concern as soon as she felt he was falling behind. He was unable to explain his practice exercises to me so there was no reinforcement at home. (Dad has no musical talent so no help coming from Dad.) At that point, I was determined to at least do everything I could think of to help him, since he was so excited about it and wanted to play so badly. I asked if I could sit in on the classes for a while so that I could see and hear what was taking place. Then we could come home and practice. She was very receptive to my idea and even seemed excited about it. She also introduced us to the person that would prove to be Trampus's "foundation for success." Her name is Gretchen Bowles and by accepting our encouragement to be firm with him, she has given him an incredible foundation. We still, today, are amazed at what Trampus has been able to accomplish through her encouragement and help.

Trampus and I would take the lessons home each day and practice. We would make flash cards to aid in learning the key signatures, the notes, and the timing. Sometimes we would battle, but no matter how tired or discouraged we became, his desire to keep on "keeping on" would bring us back on task. (I never forced him to learn anything. If it's his desire, he will pursue it with passion. Otherwise, failure is just waiting around the corner.) One of the greatest gifts given to someone with Down syndrome is their determination. The important thing we must do is to direct that determination. (This is one more example of the significance of learning discipline and authority.)

It was so amazing to watch this group of sixth graders (most of whom had never played an instrument) work together and perform a concert at Christmas. They did beautifully, and each one enjoyed the standing ovation they received! What an exciting evening seeing Trampus dressed in his tux shirt and pants and included in this group of talented students. It was well worth all the time and hard work to see our family watch Trampus perform and glow with pride.

I'm convinced that his love for performing (as well as the attention) has been one of the major forces that drives him to continue the hard work with the trumpet. The opportunity to have been a part of an excellent program that took the Laing Symphonic Band to superior ratings, not only in state competitions, but to the Grand NAI in Chattanooga, Tennessee, stimulated his appetite for perfection.

It really was neat to see him reach the level of talent that not only allowed him to keep up with his fellow band members, but to excel with them. It was no longer necessary for me to sit in on the classes, or sit in on his individual lessons. We worked together in the evenings, but that may have been for me as much as for him.

Because he has always had such a love for performing, I can remember trying to think of opportunities for him to perform. I remember hearing about the agenda for one of the Special Olympics South Carolina Mid-Winter Games. They always opened the games with "The Star-Spangled Banner". *Aha!* He could learn the national anthem on the trumpet and play at the opening ceremony. I couldn't get to Ms. Schneider quick enough. I knew there was a good chance that some of the notes might be too high, so I figured we could just drop down an octave if necessary. She was very supportive and had a friend produce a version that he could play. Everything was coming together; everyone began to get as excited as Trampus and I. Then the reality of what I had arranged began to hit me. He was going to be standing on the stage before two thousand plus people, all eyes on him, playing "The Star-Spangled Banner." My earlier *aha!* began to feel like *ugh!* Could he actually stand before everyone and still concentrate on his music? Would he be able to produce the beautiful clear tones that would come from strong air being pushed through the trumpet? I'm sure my concern was coming from the fact that I could hardly breathe at all just thinking of him there, let alone knowing the need for strong breath on his part. As usual, he stepped up to the plate and was able to "awe" the crowd with his talent and determination. My heart was beating so hard that I can't honestly say that I heard him; in fact, I found myself a bit concerned that maybe everyone was hearing my heart pound over his trumpet. He was so pleased to be a part of the program, and needless to say, we were so proud of him. I knew that this was just the beginning for him. Special Olympics South Carolina had already become a very special part of our lives. Special Olympics president, Barry Coats, and executive vice-president, Sue Maner, and all of those who work with them to help bring joy to the lives of the special needs communities of SC truly gave Trampus the platform to show people what can happen with vision, hope, and support. They have been so encouraging and are continuously looking for opportunities for Trampus to show off his "ability." They have worked diligently to take focus away from the world's eye-view of "dis" ability. Thank you guys for all you do. I'm still amazed how day in and day out, year in and year out, your love and excitement never seems to diminish.

The special needs community has several organizations that try to bring attention and acclamation to those who are an integral part of supporting the young people that may need extra attention. One of the ways this was implemented was through "The Star Award" given to people nominated by families of special needs children. We nominated Jan Holzberger for all of her time and effort. Well, I thought if we were going to have an opportunity to bring all of these people together to say thank you, how special it would be for Trampus to open the program with "The Star-Spangled Banner." I talked with Kay Ciganovic, truly a saint for the community of special people, and she was very supportive of the idea. It just so happened she had not yet printed the program, so it was settled; Trampus would open the ceremony. He did a beautiful job and truly amazed those in attendance. I think it was the first time even the Kutchers had heard him play by himself, and they were speechless. The next day, they couldn't brag enough about him. He was so excited about the accolades. The word was out: Trampus was truly a "trumpeter."

Within a few weeks of his performance, we had an opportunity to go to a RiverDogs baseball game (Charleston's semi-professional baseball team) for Special Olympics night. I thought to myself, *What a great opportunity if Trampus could play at one of the games at Joe field!* I found one of the managers that night and asked what would be the possibility of Trampus playing at one of the games. His response was definitely positive, but I would need to and was instructed to contact their program director to set up an audition. Before I knew it, I had the business card and had made the call. I explained the situation and told them about his previous performances. They set a date for him to come and audition. Here we go again: sounds great until time to produce. Trampus was all excited about the thought of playing for a baseball game and when the day arrived for the audition, he asked me to wait in the car. He and his private instructor, Gretchen Bowles, took his stand, trumpet, and music, and proceeded to the field. I waited quietly outside the gates for their return. As I saw them rounding the corner, Gretchen held a thumbs-up sign. Everyone was excited, and we were able to set the date he would play: June 6, 2002. It was a nerve-racking, but incredible experience, to see him standing on that field opening the game with "The Star-Spangled Banner." Gretchen was by his side keeping the music from blowing away. Naturally, the stands went crazy as he finished, and both he and Gretchen beamed with joy. What a great accomplishment for the two of them!

Mr. Jeremy Rohr, the band director that replaced Christina Schneider, was behind Trampus from the beginning. He encouraged him and was always ready to help. Each year the students were prompted to audition for several state competitions. I had not pursued any of these competitions until Trampus was in the eighth grade. Mr. Rohr pressed us to participate in the All-County auditions if for no other reason than for the experience. He felt that he had a good chance of being selected.

Trampus would have to know his scales by memory, play a solo that he had been given to practice, and then he would have to sight-read a piece of music he had never seen. In addition, he would be asked definitions of certain musical terms. There would be three judges in a room (hidden behind a screen). Each judge would be responsible for one of the three areas. It just so happened that the day scheduled for the audition was also the day of the Special Olympics Soccer Tournament. Fortunately, the auditions were at Cario Middle School, which was right next door to the soccer fields. He was able to play the first period of the soccer tournament and then we scooped him up for the audition.

When we arrived, the students were already backed up. The auditions were running approximately thirty minutes behind. As we sat there, we saw student after student walk out, some very quietly, some shaking their heads, and some with tears running down their cheeks. I thought to myself, *What have I done now?* Interestingly enough, Trampus was unmoved by what he saw and just sat there waiting for his turn. Suddenly, I heard his name called. Mr. Rohr had told me that he thought it would be best to let him be judged along with the others with no acknowledgement of differences. Of course, I wanted him to have any advantage he could get, but was confident that Mr. Rohr knew best. I was so nervous that I had to walk away from the area during his audition, but Vince stayed until he was through. When I thought the appropriate time had passed, I returned.

Trampus came out of the room ready to get back to his soccer. We asked him how he did, and of course his comment was "great." After the game, we came home ready to unwind from what felt like a year of activities.

I remember picking up the phone and hearing the *beep* telling us there was a message, but for some reason, I was just too tired to check. We weren't home more than an hour before the phone rang. The familiar voice of Gretchen Bowles, the very one who helped in his band career successes, was on the other end. I heard the excitement in her voice as she spoke my name. "Martha, Martha, Trampus was selected for the All-County Band!" My first thought was that I must be asleep and dreaming. But as I heard Vince saying, "What's the matter?" I knew it was real. I passed the news on to him and we both just cried. I think maybe Gretchen was doing the same. Once we regained our composure, she went on to say that although it was not absolutely final, it appeared that out of sixteen chair positions as well as eight alternates, Trampus had made sixth chair. He had received a superior rating on sight-reading! All of his hard work and his commitment to his music had paid off, and he would receive the ultimate "pat on the back." We all knew that Ms. Schneider had made this possible, and Mr. Rohr kept it going, but a great deal of the credit had to go to Gretchen who was the one person who had pressed in and worked with Trampus day after day. She was truly the one who had to show continuous patience and perseverance in teaching the skills that allowed him to read his music with such confidence, and honed his ability to count which is so important in sight-reading. We shared the joy of our "little man" and said good night. Of course, we had to talk to the man whom Trampus "wanted to be just like." I could see we had received a message from Jeremy, so I returned his call. Again, we shared the joy with Jeremy, and finally rested peacefully knowing that each of us had played a role in helping someone accomplish a desire that obviously had been placed deep inside. That banner day was one for the memory books, and proved to be just the beginning of many wonderful occasions to come!

There have been so many opportunities for Trampus to share his talent. I remember one time when Vince called and asked if I thought Trampus would be able to play a few Disney tunes (he had CDs that were "play along") for one of the elementary classes in Mt. Pleasant. The teacher had gone to school with my daughter, remembered Trampus, and had heard he played the trumpet. She had a student in her class that had Down syndrome, and thought it would be a great opportunity to show all of the students what can happen with a vision and hard work. Of course we did it, and once again, it was so much fun to see the smiling faces, but this time, the little children were "rockin'" with the music. The word got out that he had a five- to ten-minute repertoire so he was asked to play during the lunch break of a Special Education Conference for The Charleston County School District, as well as performing for his former alma mater, Whitesides Elementary PTA meeting. He continues to play for many of the Special Olympics Games and ceremonies. He has played in many different venues such as Central Park in New York City opening the National Buddy Walk; the The Star Spangled Banner for basketball games for The Citadel College, Charleston Southern

University, The College of Charleston, as well as the University of South Carolina. I remember one of those games when USC was playing Florida and USC had not beaten them in quite a while. The stands were full. I was a nervous wreck so Vince agreed to go with Trampus to the waiting area. We were told they would bring him on the court ten minutes prior to the game. I was sitting in my seat watching the time and began to panic when I suddenly realized Vince and Trampus were not in the designated spot. It was almost time to come out and they were no where to be found. Right as my knees began to buckle and I thought I might be sick, Trampus walked on to the court. Later Vince explained that right before the ten-minute deadline, Trampus decided he needed to make a nature call. He informed his father there was no waiting. Wow! Ten-thousand people waiting while he was in the potty. I'm always amazed how he seems to perform his best in the largest arenas. He did a wonderful job producing a standing ovation and the applause was deafening. When he finished playing, up went his arms to pump up the crowd. It worked! The crowd went crazy. I still say it was the excitement he stirred up that day that gave USC an incredible win in the last three seconds of the game. He played both "The Star-Spangled Banner" and "Taps" at several of the Law Enforcement Torch Run Kick-offs. These ceremonies not only serve as the opening of the Torch Run, but they honor law enforcement officers who lost their lives in the line of duty. He continues to participate in their events even today. He has been given the honor of an invitation to play "Amazing Grace" at the funeral services of three of our very dear friends, Bill Kulseth, Rebecca Kuther's mother, Robert Lever, as well as Trampus's grandfather. We were so proud of him and there were truly no dry eyes. One of the most memorable and extraordinary invitations came from the Superintendent of Education for South Carolina. We received a call from Gretchen asking if he would play for one of the State Board of Education's meetings. He would be playing "America," "The Star-Spangled Banner," "Amazing Grace," and the solo he played for the All-County Band audition. Of course, he accepted and it was very impressive when we arrived in Columbia to find a parking place in the front of the building with a printed sign "Reserved for the Musician for The State Board Meeting."

It was difficult to see the completion of another major time period for Trampus—middle school. We had such a wonderful three years at Laing, and it was very tough to walk away from the security of being known and appreciated, and from the fun of all the successes we had enjoyed. I remember having the same feelings when we were saying our good-byes to Whitesides. What I learned was that each change that comes to us opens up another opportunity to see him (along with myself) grow, mature, and continue to fulfill the purpose for which we were created.

HIGH SCHOOL

We began our talks at Wando High School. We wanted to help them get to know Trampus a little better before school started the following year, so we planned a visit. We were looking at our options in the programs available in order to select the one that would provide the necessary atmosphere for him to succeed. Of course, the school was involved in the discussion, and I listened carefully and then helped guide their thinking so that when the final decision was made, we would all be in agreement: working together for his success. I could feel the excitement of the parents of the special needs children at Laing who would be following us in the next few years. I can still sense the pressure that comes with being one of the ones helping to pave the way on this road we're all walking down, but I also know that my confidence comes from the same light that has guided us through each door.

When Trampus was in the seventh grade at Laing, the attendance clerk decided to resign and go into the classroom as a teaching assistant. It was pointed out that since I already spent a good bit of time at Laing, I might as well apply for the position and get paid for being there. Good plan, but my first response was negative. I had become accustomed to the freedom of working at my convenience with our family business, and I wasn't sure I was ready to be tied down to an eight-hour workday, five days a week. However, it became apparent that we were going to have trouble with insurance for Trampus when we found it necessary to change our health insurance company. If I went to work for Laing which was a state agency, Trampus would automatically be covered.

Once again, I could see our needs were being met and what a great way for me to be available to advocate and help should Trampus need it.

As our time at Laing drew to a close, I thought about applying for a position at Wando High School where Trampus would be attending. I would be able to continue following Trampus and help as needed. After talking with Lou Cothran, the director of special education at that time, about that possibility, her response was "maybe it's time to allow him to move around without a net." *Ugh!* But maybe she was right. At least I was in the school system and close enough to be there quickly if necessary. Okay, I'm good with that. Then the call came from Lucy Beckham, the principal at Wando. She wanted to talk to me about a position in the front office. When I mentioned my discussion with Lou, Lucy felt it only made sense to follow him and then I could choose to get involved or step aside. Confusion…do I follow and stay close or step back and begin to stand on the sidelines? Thank goodness I have always been confident that whether my decisions are good or bad, I can count on God's Word that promises He can work all things together for good for those who love Him, and He continuously gives me cause to trust Him.

By the time I had my next conversation with Lou, she had changed her mind and agreed with Lucy that it would be better for Trampus and Wando if I was there. I talked with Trampus and he agreed, so it was final. I would become a "Wando Warrior" with him. Trampus and I felt like we had already had a little practice at being "warriors."

We were very fortunate that the school music community, particularly the band programs, worked closely together in Mt. Pleasant. As a result, the word was already out about Trampus and his trumpet, so we met with Lou and Mr. Scott Rush, the band director, to determine Trampus's role in the band at the high school level. I could sense his excitement, as well as his enthusiasm. All of my concerns began to disappear as I listened to his soft reassuring voice. There was not a doubt in my mind that he had been listening to the same "inner man" voice because everything he was saying about what he envisioned for Trampus was one with mine. There was no hesitancy in his desire to have Trampus become a part of the Wando High School band program, and he and Sean McGrew, the assistant band director, had already made plans for the marching band. *Yuk!* I had "mustered" up most of my faith just to see Trampus play the trumpet. Now we were going to have to memorize a minimum of three songs along with approximately eight minutes of marching around in a specific pattern on the field.

Sean was the percussion instructor and had offered to have him start off his marching band experience with the percussionists. He had plans to work with him on the marimbas and several other instruments. He and Scott had agreed that there was a good bit more "downtime" and since the percussion area (except for the drums) didn't have to march, he could concentrate on the music.

I could tell when Trampus and I talked about Wando and the marching band he was excited but nervous. He wanted to be a part of the band, but really didn't care about trying to march. Once I explained that he would not have to learn the routine and play while he marched, he was eager to get started.

Our life at Wando would begin about three weeks before school actually started. He would attend "rookie" band camp one week before the full band came to prepare for the competitions that would culminate in the State Marching Band Championship in November. *Gotcha!* No problem. What time did I need to have him at the school? Nine o'clock. No problem. Then what time would I need to come and get him? Nine o'clock…no, must be some confusion…I meant pick him up! They responded nine o'clock *in the evening!* I still marvel today at the commitment and endurance of band students. We would see the football team come and go as these students learned that particular year's production. What a work ethic and love for music! That time together, I am convinced, is what produces the "family" atmosphere, and results in the oneness that takes over among the students.

I could not imagine that Trampus would be able to stay out there in the heat for that long, let alone learn what was needed. My first thought was that he usually requires more time than others and there wasn't any more "time" available. *Whew!* Once again I found that when we discover something he wants, he will not let go until he is able to do it.

Sean McGrew and the percussion students literally embraced him. They became as determined for him, as he was, to learn what was required for Trampus's part. Sean actually wrote in the music for Trampus's part and did it based on what he saw Trampus could do. Now keep in mind Sean was doing all this while preparing his group for competition. I don't think we will ever really know how very big a part Sean, Scott, and all of the band family have played in the triumphs Trampus has enjoyed. I'm sure I will never know the many challenges they conquered without me. I do remember one time when we were on our way home and Trampus seemed down. I can't remember why, but I think he had to be reprimanded for something he did or did not do at band camp. I began to reinforce his need to listen and obey as I am so capable of doing, and doing it with a vengeance. As I looked over at him and our eyes met, I could see a tear. He looked away and said, "I just want to be like everyone else, Mom." *Ugh!* Sometimes it is so difficult for me to know when to be quiet. Thank goodness for the love, compassion, and sincerity that he experienced while a part of Wando High School, especially the music family. It's so amazing to be able to step back and objectively see the relationships that grow from differences. It's awesome to see people learn to embrace and overcome differences rather than continue to not understand or just hold on to fears. What a joy to see fear turn to love: first in my own life, then others as they allow themselves to be exposed to the unknown. What an opportunity to learn to grow in the skills of life. It saddens me to think how many times these opportunities are missed because of the hardness of hearts. I better understand now when people say, "God gives these children to special people." Yes he does…to those who, like me, need most to learn unconditional love and need to learn to be selfless. Thankfully, everyone doesn't have to "birth" and take on this opportunity in the natural or full time, but rather can experience it on a part-time basis. I am becoming more and more convinced that God has called Vince and me to work and live this out before others, trusting Him to guide us so that many will learn the enjoyment that can come from what may "feel" or "appear" to be a very discouraging and scary experience as a parent.

The band became our lifeline and was a large part of life at Wando (except for his participation in the drama department headed by Ms. Selina May which I will talk about a little further into my story.) Because I was employed by the school, I was able to take time from work as a chaperone and travel with the band when needed. I believed it was important for me to be with him on these trips because I had come to understand that the most difficult part of life for people with special needs and those around them is to be able to interact. It can be difficult learning how to see each other's role in not just communicating, but enjoying an active, viable relationship. We still, today, find that to be one of our biggest challenges. By Trampus growing up in the "inclusion" world, there were usually always "facilitators" whether in the form of teachers, staff, or even students. There were always those students around that either Trampus grew up with, or new ones that had a tender heart. Many times I would find that these students had already had an opportunity to be around people who were "different." As a result, Trampus had little practice in carrying the major role in communicating.

When the days and hours of practice began to wind down, and the time to perform in the competitions came, Trampus and I had pretty much learned the "ins and outs" of band life. Many of the parents that were the leaders in the Booster Club were former band members themselves, so they usually kept the operation going smoothly. The program required a tremendous volunteer force. Trips had to be planned, buses arranged, hotel accommodations booked, food and drinks provided not only for regular meals, but for practice times in between. One thing I was sure of: too many people doing too much, too quickly, to try and make sure Trampus was in uniform, in the right place, and at the right time. It just couldn't have happened if I had not been able to be there.

Wando High School's music department is absolutely the best there is! Many college programs envy the successes Wando has consistently enjoyed, which could fill a book. We were humbled and honored to see the time and energy this incredible group was willing to give to a student with special needs. Their hard work with Trampus gave him the tools he needed to be successful in so many other areas of his life. The confidence he developed from their influence and efforts will continue to follow him throughout his entire life. He was awarded the Esprit de Corps Award (the common spirit existing in the members of a group inspiring enthusiasm, devotion, and strong regard for the honor of the group) his senior year and it sits very proudly on our living room table right next to his "Honor Band" award he received while at Laing Middle School. Scott decided to establish a "Wall of Fame" in the band area and Trampus received the honor of being the first student to begin filling that space. *Wow!* Just the other day Trampus and Vince were shopping and several Wando band students were fundraising in the front of the store. Trampus approached to purchase a card and although he has not attended Wando since 2008, the student recognized him from his picture on the "Wall of Fame."

Once school started, the band rehearsals continued, but they were now only two evenings each week from 5:00 p.m. to 9:00 p.m. All of this band time had helped him to become comfortable with his "Wando" family. It also gave him an opportunity to learn how to "be still for long periods," especially since Wando's class schedule included four ninety-minute classes each day.

Concert band made up one of those classes. One was English, one math, and one PE. His English and math were self-contained. Because students in the self-contained program are unable to complete the requirements needed for receiving Carnegie credits, they receive a certificate of attendance. Up until now, because they did not receive the high school diploma, they were not eligible to pursue college. That was one of the main reasons we chose to concentrate and focus on his music. We had no idea the doors that could and would open to non-diploma graduates.

The first year at Wando was spent learning the academia "ropes." There were around two thousand students on campus and six hundred of those were a part of Trampus's graduating class. The "exceptional" students, as referred to now, had the opportunity to select elective courses such as PE, art, band, drama, etc. After that first year, I began to look more closely at some of those "extra classes" available at Wando. I saw a couple that caught my eye in computer science and creative writing. I requested permission for Trampus to take these courses. It was understood that he would be auditing the class so there would not be pressure or extra work on the teacher. We were always looking for opportunities to try and put him in as "normal" an environment as possible in order to help develop his social skills, and secondly to survey for areas of strength. I am convinced that although Trampus was unable to grasp all that was offered in these classes, what he did gain is influencing what he is able to do today.

One incredible experience for all of us came when Trampus informed me he was going to take algebra. Since math had never been a subject he was able to grasp and he had never shown interest, I was naturally surprised and curious. Why this interest? I found out that he had been going to Joe Kutcher's classroom before school and asking Joe to help him with algebra. (Joe had joined Wando and taught the engineering classes which also included math. Joe has since passed away and has left a void that will never be filled.) He began to work with Trampus without mentioning it to me. It always amazes me how excellent teachers are able to produce a love for their subject out of the students that have exposure to them. Trampus continued to persist in taking algebra even to the point of checking out a book on algebra from the library. Joe and I discussed the possibility, and he talked with one of the teachers that taught an algebra class for students that needed reinforcement. Her name was Jennifer Smith Houston and she became the "star" in Trampus's eyes. He took her class and it was love at first sight for the two of them. She encouraged him and bragged on his areas of strength. She would give him the encouragement he needed when he became frustrated because of his inability to follow along. She told me there were some things he grasped better than other students. She was constantly looking for ways to help him in the weak areas. It was a wonderful experience for Trampus and he still talks about taking "algebra" even today.

Trampus had never been particularly interested in coloring or working with crafts. I always enjoyed it and would come up with projects to do with him and our grandchildren. Within a short time, Trampus would have haphazardly "completed" his, while the others meticulously went about finalizing and perfecting their artistic design. This helped me to make the decision to stay away from the art classes. I believe one of the areas most difficult for teachers or anyone trying to share something they love is to have to try to teach or work with others who do not care or have an interest in that same love.

I did know from past experiences that he loved "acting" and "performing" so naturally we signed him up for drama.

I'm astounded by the people that have come into our lives and put themselves in the middle of Trampus's learning experience. This is such a confirmation that when we expect and look for the positive, it will always present itself through others with that same expectation. It happened when we signed Trampus up for Drama I, II, and III. Normally, I immediately put myself in the middle of the situation as to advocate and press for what I believe needs to happen. This time, with band and work, I just didn't have a chance to put in my usual "two cents." Boy was that good 'cause the last thing that Salina and Ryan May needed was my input. Here were two wonderful people who had a heart to take what they love and reproduce it in someone else. They knew that if they needed me, I would be there, but otherwise, they took him under their wing and off they went. I would love to be able to say that I played a large role in his acting experience, but I was the transporter and attendee in the world of drama. Trampus loved working with the lighting and sound, but Selina kept pressing him to allow the part of him that loved performing to come out in his acting.

It was incredible to watch the insecurity that was there in the beginning come to a culmination of seeing him perform in *A Midsummer Night's Dream*, *To Kill a Mockingbird*, and *Charlie and the Chocolate Factory* during his three years in drama. Also the honor of receiving an invitation to join the Thespian Society and to participate in the National Individual Events Showcase at Converse College, South Carolina.

After three years of working with Trampus, Selina came to me and asked if I would be comfortable with a skit that she wanted Trampus to learn and present at the Thespian Festival. She wanted him to perform a portion from *Flowers for Algernon*. I knew nothing about it but she went on to explain that it was the story of a mentally challenged young man who would have the opportunity to be given a pill that would make him "normal." She didn't want to offend me but felt that the greatest part of performing comes when it is closest to the person you are. Of course I had complete confidence in her request and said, "Absolutely." I offered to help with memorization if she would work on everything else. I made the trip with the drama club and marveled at all of the talent among these high school students.

Since I agreed to get Trampus to his judging room, we set out for the scheduled performance that morning. I could tell he was nervous, but I fought the hardest at not exposing my own fears. I'm going to learn one day that he seems to flourish when the pressure comes. As the judges called his number to come up to the front of the class, I truly thought I might get sick. I was in trouble. I couldn't leave. I was in the middle of the room surrounded by people with no place to run. *Ouch!* I looked down and tried to quiet my heart. Then, I heard my son reciting the dialogue with such peace and with so much emotion; I could feel the first tear begin to well up in my eyes. Then, without any ability to stop them, they flowed down my cheeks. As I looked up, I was not alone. Most in the room were experiencing the same. When he finished, he politely bowed to the judges, turned to us in the room with a confident smile, bowed, and proceeded to come sit next to me. *Wow!*

Selina found me later in the morning and was so excited but I couldn't make out what she was trying to tell me. She was a judge for another group so had little time to talk, but tried to tell me something about his being one of the ten performances, out of approximately three hundred, selected to perform on the last day before all of the students, faculty members, and judges at the festival, a packed auditorium. What she later explained to me was that the judges and selection committee felt that it was imperative for teachers and students to see what can be accomplished by anyone with a heart to succeed. That afternoon in the Converse College auditorium, Trampus stood up and, I believe, gave the performance of his life. It was probably the best opportunity for advocating since he was up on stage, with everyone's undivided attention sharing his heart.

Selina and Ryan, thank you for taking your God-given talent, your love and compassion, and using it to touch so many lives. We miss you both!

I believe because so much of Trampus's life was surrounded by adults as well as much older siblings, he tended to search out that environment. Although he did not enjoy the physical part of PE at the high school level, he loved to interact with the coaches. Each one played a tremendous role in helping Trampus learn to be a part of something! He always loved that. But one man who stood out among all the coaches was the athletic director and head football coach, Bob Hayes. Boy, did Trampus love that man. Coach would allow Trampus to come in and discuss "plays" that should be used for the next football game. Trampus would ask for advice on…well, only Bob, Trampus, and God really know. I do know that Coach Hayes confirmed our efforts in trying to teach Trampus the importance of respect for authority and commitment to do what is right. We found out through Trampus that Coach Hayes would be coaching the North South Football game. He also informed us that Coach Hayes would give him tickets if we could go. I watched as Trampus looked his dad in the eyes and begged, "Dad, please, can we go to Myrtle Beach and watch Coach Hayes." Needless to say, Vince agreed to take him, so Trampus tucked away his tickets and counted off the days until the game. The next school day after the game, Coach Hayes found me and told me how much he appreciated Trampus coming to the game. He went on to explain to me that this was the first game that his family had not been able to attend. His wife had been sick, and so he was at the game alone. He said that as he was feeling somewhat saddened by their absence, he heard this voice yelling, "Coach Hayes! Coach Hayes!" He looked up in the stands and there at the rail was Trampus, smiling big as ever, waving and offering him the big thumbs-up. What a moment for the two of them. Thank you, Bob, for loving our son and for being a part of our "success" story!

Because of their inclusion opportunities and successes, Trampus and Trista Kutcher were nominated by their Exceptional Education teachers at Wando and selected by Charleston County School District, along with another young man, to be considered for an International Awards Program established in 1981 by The Foundation for Exceptional Children. The program was established to acknowledge the achievements of children and youth with disabilities; overcome barriers caused by public misconceptions and to encourage children and youth with disabilities to seek their highest potential; and increase public awareness of the abilities, aspirations and personal qualities of people with disabilities. We were asked to put together all of his accomplishments and it was sent to the national selection committee for review. We found out that spring, that the three Charleston County students had been selected for each of their divisions out of approximately three thousand students worldwide. Trampus received the award for his accomplishments in music, Trista for athletics, and the other student for his work ethic. The students and their families were all invited to Louisville, Kentucky. It was very moving to see each of them receive a bronze statue and a letter from President Bush and the First Lady. What a wonderful experience and honor for all of the Charleston County School District, the community, and the families.

As a result of Trampus playing his trumpet all around the community, he had several opportunities to meet the mayor of our town, Harry Hallman. We were so excited and honored when we received the call that the mayor wanted to present Trampus with the "Key to the City." Mayor Hallman has since passed away but his memory will be with us forever.

Another great opportunity for advocating while Trampus was at Wando came when the National Down Syndrome Society asked for members throughout the United States to send a picture that emphasized an example of inclusion in everyday life. Several people encouraged us to send a picture of Trampus with his trumpet. We selected a picture that included him with several other trumpet players in their band uniform warming up for a half-time performance. We sent it in and were contacted that summer that his picture had been selected, and he would be on the huge Auditron in Times Square. I couldn't leave it at that…but when they called to tell us he had been selected, I had to mention that he was able to play "The Star-Spangled Banner" and maybe it would be great if he played for the day of the "Buddy Walk" in Central Park. Of course they agreed, so it was set. He would open the walk with his trumpet. You'd think that it would get to be "old hat" after a while, but I still have to settle my nerves and concentrate on seeing him play with success each time he performs. Our local news anchor, Dean Stephens, who did a special report on Trampus's life, was very excited for him. Dean would not be able to travel to New York but asked that we record the event for WCIV Television an affiliate of ABC.

The selected pictures were shown as a slideshow the day before the National Down Syndrome Buddy Walk kick off. What an experience to be standing in Times Square looking up and seeing Trampus come across that huge screen. His sister was able to be with us, and all we could do was stand there amazed as we watched all of these people, some standing, some walking by, but most staring at these precious people coming across the screen.

Another incredible moment came for Trampus when the student council advisement teacher, Michelle Smith, suggested that Trampus consider entering the "Mr. Wando Contest." She pointed out that he could play his trumpet for his talent and stressed the fun that the guys had in preparing. We were all excited and he selected a song to perform. The boys were put in groups and had to prepare a skit. Here was another opportunity for Trampus to interact with other "guys" in a social environment. Yet another chance to be a part and "fit in." He needed an escort for that evening and he already knew who he would ask. Her name was Jessie Gravino, and she was a very special person in Trampus's life while at Wando, and was excited when he asked her. She is very sensitive to the special needs community because she has a brother, Zack, with Down syndrome and is also a friend of Trampus. It was a very exciting evening, and he did a tremendous job with his trumpet. The judges made their decision and everyone was brought on stage. I listened as they slowly announced the winners of each category: best talent, most cordial, Mr. Senior, Mr. Junior, Mr. Sophomore, Mr. Freshman. I could see Trampus's face as he listened and watched each young man walk to the center to receive his award. I wondered, *What is he thinking right now? Does he even realize what is happening?* The anticipation was coming to an end. The time had come to announce the winner of the 2008 Mr. Wando contest…and suddenly the announcer called Trampus Hoover…William Sunday Trampus Hooover. What emotions flowed from that auditorium! For some of the boys, I'm sure there was disappointment in losing, but many of the people shared the excitement of such an incredible award for the special needs community. (Michelle Smith told me afterwards that the judges had assured her their decision was based on the required criteria and he had won outright.) Word spread quickly and Trampus found himself in the middle of the "limelight" enjoying every moment. Even to the extent that the next morning he stood in the front of the school greeting each incoming student wearing his crown and sash.

There is a wonderful organization in the tri-county area, The Down Syndrome Association of the Lowcountry (DSAL). While we were not active when Trampus was younger, we became more involved during his high school years. As I mentioned before, we had determined that he needed to be more involved with the special needs community and this was a perfect avenue for that. The social aspects of life with Down syndrome is probably the most problematic. Rebecca Kutcher felt that it was important to establish an advocacy group with DSAL and asked if Trampus would serve as the first chairperson (I would serve as co-chair). We accepted and have many wonderful memories of that period of time. We scheduled the meetings for Friday evenings and it would include a cook-out, maybe a movie, games outside, and we spent time helping them to understand advocating for themselves. No mentors; just each other learning communications skills within their own community. The parents were invited if they wished and we would socialize as well.

Our desire was to provide a means of learning to interact with each other in order to provide a social life after their graduation from school. Anything else that they gained would just be a plus. Trampus served his time and then passed the baton to Trista Kutcher. It was difficult for us to continue due to a change of meeting schedule and the focus seemed to be moving more toward independent learning rather than social interaction. Again, our real interest was to help him learn to be a part of a group regardless of the make-up of that group. We wanted him to learn how to make conversation without "outside" help. This is still an important issue for us today, and we are encouraged as we see the patience of the community around us as he matures.

COLLEGE

What an incredible time Trampus experienced in high school. Our expectations have always been high and we have always known that each day that comes is an opportunity to see the marvelous works of our Creator, but even with that attitude, I couldn't have asked for more for Trampus. In fact, there are times that I just can't even grasp what he has accomplished.

The positive part of Trampus's high school life was the incredible role modeling he received particularly through his music. He has always seen himself as one of "them." The negative is that there has been little self-advocating required and even less time spent with others with special needs. His comfort zone was being established, excluding others like himself. Once again, I can see the importance of balance. There was a role reversal being established and we didn't realize it. Trampus, at times, was doing the very thing we were always looking for ways to avoid. We have asked the "normal" community to accept Trampus and most have, yet here he was having difficulty accepting those like himself. Because of all he continues to accomplish, it is very easy to become all about Trampus: how smart, what a hard worker, how talented he is. Through our advocating, promotion, and protection, Trampus has experienced very few failures which I believe as of today has proven both good and counter-productive. While it has given him a great deal of self-confidence and self-worth, many of our lessons in life come as a result of our failures. Many times our difficulties can help us mature and bring us to a place of selflessness, along with the ability to "overcome" those difficulties.

Here we were, at the end of a wonderful period of time in his life, and now we had to move on.

We have wonderful friends that have always embraced Trampus, but there is one couple that has always been drawn to Trampus and he to them. It was kind of like they were the "hip" mom and dad not the "stuffy don't do this and be sure and do that" mom and dad. It started when they surprised us by their moving from Charlotte, North Carolina, and buying the house right behind ours. Robert and Carolyn Lever truly became mentors and provided reinforcement for decisions made when Trampus didn't like or agree with them. They also helped me see times when I needed to back off. I think the closeness that they enjoyed with Trampus was because of their ability to love unconditionally like he does. It was very difficult for all of us when Robert passed away, but his memory is etched in our hearts and I can still hear him calling my son's name.

As a result of their involvement in a local faith community church, Seacoast Church, I began to wonder if this might be an opportunity to become a part of the faith community, as well as help Trampus focus on others. He was receiving no formal religious exposure so we knew that left a definite void in this area of his life. Although our hope that he would be able to become a part of the young adult group did not come to fruition, he was able to help with the technology department crew. These volunteers would work sound and lighting for the Kids Coast. Trampus had been involved in the "technical world" through his involvement in drama and the many productions performed, so this was a good match. They were wonderful with him and he loved being a part of the team.

We enjoyed our time at Seacoast but found ourselves missing some of the traditions and fulfillments received through the Eucharist. Although we first believed Seacoast would help Trampus, I now believe it played a role in helping us to see God's desire for forgiveness and oneness, and to let go of injuries that only divide. As a result, we decided to visit a Catholic church near our home, and even though we were thankful for our time at Seacoast, we felt St. Benedict's was where we needed to be.

As I had mentioned before, college for Trampus was never in the picture; so now what. We knew he would be able to come and help out with our family business but was that really what he wanted to do? Didn't he need an opportunity to have a say in how he would spend his workdays?

We have a business that has provided us a wonderful relationship with Charleston Southern University, and an opportunity to discuss the possibility of Trampus attending the school. They did not offer the LIFE (Learning Is For Everyone) program but after meeting with the appropriate people, much prayer and I'm sure the prayers of those at CSU involved in this endeavor, Trampus was offered a hybrid curriculum. It included private trumpet lessons, Concert Band, Marching Band, Pep Band, Beginning Piano, and Theory and Music Appreciation. He worked very hard and accomplished a great deal. Boy did we plow through the Theory class. We realized how difficult the class was going to be and even more difficult since I was unable to sit in on the lectures. Thank goodness the professor was incredible, and the university recorded the class so that Trampus and I could see and listen to the lectures at home. We both learned a great deal. He loved the piano keyboard class and again worked really hard. He still enjoys just sitting down and playing from his music books. He was not only a part of the marching band but even learned to march while playing his trumpet. He was able to march at the University of Miami vs. CSU in Miami. The only problem, they were not equipped for him to be able to stay on campus and get the "real" campus life experience. They tried to find a way, but couldn't make it happen. They just were unable to accept that kind of liability. Although he has many fond memories, we knew this was not really what we were trying to accomplish. We were trying to give him an opportunity to begin to learn how to function without us being right there in the forefront. We wanted him to have an opportunity to begin to be his own advocate. We knew this would be a tremendous challenge but we also felt that with our help, he could become his own best help.

As mentioned earlier, we had been hearing about a program that would provide students with special needs an opportunity to attend college and live on campus. The National Down Syndrome had provided a grant for colleges to help establish the program and, with the hard work of many people in our community, several of the state colleges took on the challenge of providing the "LIFE Program" on their campuses. "Learning is for Everyone" was put in place within a couple of years at Clemson University, University of South Carolina, and Coastal Carolina University.

As we thought through the next step for Trampus, we took notice of the program at Coastal Carolina. The Clemson program was a no go mainly because of the location. Too far away! USC did not offer "housing" so the only real option for us was CCU. Coastal seemed to have everything in place, and not only that, we have a house in Myrtle Beach that we rent during the summer months, but is usually available during the winter months. In the meantime, I had an opportunity to talk with Scott Rush about the band program at CCU and he knew the director. Perfect! Trampus not only would have an opportunity to learn independence, but could possibly be involved in the band as well. We would have a place to stay if there was something happening on campus that required our presence.

There are advantages and disadvantages to being in the forefront of a movement. (This was Coastal Carolina University's first year). Many accolades come as a result of stepping out and being the first to accomplish something. At the same time, you miss the perfection that can only be learned through trial and error. A friend, and expert, on including those in the special needs community says it takes four years to instill a culture.

We set up an appointment to look at the campus and the program that would be starting up at Coastal Carolina University in Myrtle Beach, South Carolina. Our biggest concern was the fact that we would be sending Trampus away from home when he had never spent more than a few days away from us, and even then, he was with one of the family members. His initial reaction was "no thanks." When we discussed the possibility of his being a part of the band, his attitude began to change.

We also made an appointment for Trampus to meet the band director, and discuss his role in their program. This would be the band's first experience with a special needs student, but they were willing to allow him to participate.

After meeting with the director of the program, the registrar, the security department, and housing, and discussing the vision that CCU had for this program, things seemed to be falling in place, and it appeared that Trampus may be heading off to college for the 2009 fall semester.

Initially, the program was set up for Trampus to be on campus seven days a week with the opportunity to come home on holidays and special occasions. The plan included mentors that would be with the students helping them to get around and adapt to college life. In the beginning, the arrangement was for a dorm of four bedrooms with a community kitchen, bathroom, and living area. One of the four students would be an RA, one would be a special needs student, and the remaining two would be regular students.

We were really excited about the way things were coming together. The campus was just beautiful. In our eyes it was the perfect size and everyone involved was excited about the new program.

When I thought my days of college preparation were over, here I was shopping for "dorm" needs. We arrived on "move in" day and were disappointed to find out that instead of one "LIFE" student, two freshman mentors, and an RA, there were two "LIFE" students, one mentor, and the RA. Rather than coming home on special occasions only (an encouragement given us at enrollment not to visit too often), we were expected to pick him up each Friday at 1:00 p.m., and not return before 6:00 p.m. on Sunday evening.

Suddenly, what we thought would be the college experience developed into no independent movement or independent participation on campus. At that point, we were told that as the students learned the "ins and outs" of the campus, they would be allowed to move around with more freedom. At least we knew he had the marching band so that would give him some independence.

After the fact, we realized we should have been more aggressive in participating in the transformation from home to college life. No one knew Trampus or his uniqueness because this was not a community where he grew up. He presented himself well, but was not accustomed to making his own decisions. We accepted the request to step back. Unfortunately, the first band trip off campus, Trampus got separated from the group. They were able to call him on his phone and find his location, but it was very upsetting for them.

After a meeting with the band director, we asked if there might be a student in the band that we could pay to help with their expenses in return for making sure Trampus was transported to and from rehearsals and band functions. Thank goodness we were able to make the arrangements and to overcome that problem.

Needless to say, Trampus had some real adjustments to undergo because of the structure he had grown up with and the lack of decision making required of him. The best thing that came from this experience was to find his strengths but more importantly, his weaknesses. Again, I think, had we been included more in the transition time at Coastal and if we had been able to participate in his course selections, the outcome might have been different.

After the end of the first year, nothing had changed. What started out as independence ended up for us, a hybrid institutionalization, and we were not allowed to be in the decision making process. The students still had to be picked up on Friday and returned at the designated time on Sunday. While Trampus loved his time at Coastal, and many wonderful people involved with Coastal Carolina, we began to question if this was really accomplishing what we had intended.

We were especially concerned that he was losing his opportunity to be involved with his music, which had always been a very important part of his life. Marching band only lasted two months, and according to his schedule, second semester would have no music classes. We explained that if he was not able to take trumpet his second year, we would have to consider pulling him out.

We were told that they would work out his trumpet class for his sophomore year and it would be one class a week. The first problem that arose was the fact that he could not practice his trumpet in the dorm room. They could not arrange a mentor to walk with him to the practice room in the band building and would not allow him to walk over by himself. Taking a class once a week without practice served no purpose. Obviously, the LIFE program was not interested in encouraging his music and actually was discouraging it.

We finally had to resign ourselves to the fact that he actually had less independence here than when he was home moving around on campus at Wando as well as Charleston Southern University. We had simply given up our control to an environment we weren't sure about and certainly not in agreement with decisions on the "how to" of life. Trampus completed the fall semester of his sophomore year at Coastal Carolina and came home. We were all disappointed that it did not turn out as we thought it would but, again, the one thing that we did get out of it was seeing the effects of Trampus out from under our thumbs. We began to see how his need for recognition and praise had taken a life of its own, and he was going to need to learn how to decrease and help those around him to increase. Trampus had definitely matured during his time at CCU.

Here we were once again examining the "what next." A funny story that occurred at this time with Trampus happened as a result of a conversation with my daughter. She's always had that "mother" instinct with Trampus, but has always been a good listener and waited before offering her thoughts and suggestions concerning him. When she heard we were bringing him home from school, she called me. She and her husband, Mark, had talked and thought maybe they had a good suggestion for Trampus. (Trampus always goes to their home in Florida for at least a week or two each summer.) She thought maybe it would be worth considering having him live with them in Florida and visit us a week or two each summer. *What?* My heart dropped to my feet with just the thought. I couldn't even speak. Was she serious? Her reasoning was he could work in their community (everyone had grown to love him during his visits) and several of her children were still in school living at home, so there was always something going on. She asked that I at least discuss the possibility with her dad. Well, with a heavy heart but respect for her request, I mentioned it, and he shot back at me without a second of time passing, "You tell her to get her own 'Downs' child." We all laughed and I still chuckle when I remember the look on his face.

In every success story there is a foundational piece that allows the structure to grow and stand firm. God established that foundation in Trampus through his grandmother. To those who know her well, she's "Gommy," the only Clemson fan in a family of University of South Carolina fans. We're sure her blood runs orange. It is difficult to see the two of them as separates, and all that we have enjoyed with Trampus would not have been possible without her. She has been his mentor, his teacher, his confidante, and his strongest supporter. She could see the stress of the start-up of a self-owned business and made herself available to cover for us when the business demanded it.

If we had to travel, she would be here to see that his school work was completed, that he ate properly, and got to the scheduled activity of the day. She has been the unending force that keeps Trampus and me pressing on. If I became tired or discouraged, she would pick up the baton and begin to run. She would sense the time to let go and I was able to continue the race.

I can see her in my mind's eye, sitting with him, the two of them, repeating the nursery rhymes that he loved so. Watching her read to him book after book until he would either move on to another adventure or fall asleep on her lap.

They would work puzzles until both of them could put them together blindfolded. You could find them sitting together intently working, each with their own word-search book. What a beautiful sight to see him sit at his grandmother's feet (just turned ninety-eight at this writing) and share their hearts with each other.

I have truly learned that when God gives you a gift (and His Word tells us that children are a gift), He provides all that is needed to enjoy that gift. My mother-in-law has been one of the invaluable tools that His Word promises, and for that, I thank Him daily.

My mother and father organized and led the Junior Civitan Clubs in South Carolina for many years. Although my mother died when Trampus was very young, my father was able to better appreciate the hard work of these young club members who help raise money for research for people with special needs. I'm sure he never realized the impact that would be felt by his own family as a result of the hard work of these young people. Trampus was able to participate in some of those functions and I believe not only enjoyed being with the young people, but gave many of them motivation and encouragement for their hard work in helping others and, of course, he has always enjoyed "showing off" his granddaddy. Dad continuously took every opportunity to inform others about his special "gift" that came in the package of his grandson. Because of my father's natural love for young people and the importance he placed on building character and compassion in each of them, Trampus provided a platform for him to carry his message throughout the teenage community. What a blessing it was to be able to call him when I felt the load was heavy and to hear his cheerful voice encouraging me to take the next step in enjoying the changes Trampus was producing in each of us! Although Dad is no longer here to call on, I can sense his love and encouragement within me, and I draw from it daily.

There is tremendous pressure today that tries to dictate the definition of success and failure. It pushes visual images, material accomplishments, and unfortunately, uses the mind (or the computer) of the individual as its power base.

There is a purpose and opportunity to every experience and decision put before us: success or failure. We're told many times that all of the situations involving our past and the circumstances around us today will determine the outcome of our lives. This is just not true! I believe that what is in us will determine the results. Some people, as a result of the environment they have been exposed to, may have a more difficult time in making these decisions, but each of us has been given the free will and ability to determine the criteria we will use to make that decision. The One who created us and set the "DNA" within us has provided information in His Last Will and Testament (The Bible), which allows us to renew our minds so that we can accomplish the purpose for which we were created. We are able to tap into that communication process by a simple prayer request to have the things of God opened up to us so that we are able to know Him and His Ways.

The physical brain is where our mind (our thoughts—intellect) is housed and is the vehicle we use to communicate with the world around us. However, there is a part of us that exists beyond our thoughts and intellect and I like to refer to it as the "inner man." Not only is the inner man (conscience) where we communicate with our Creator, but also allows communication within ourselves. It can be used to help make decisions that guide us while operating in our physical bodies. This complexity within an individual is proven in the fact that a body can be kept alive even when the brain is considered dead.

This explains the ability of a person to experience two emotions at one time, i.e., I must have this piece of candy, while at the same time reasoning that I really shouldn't eat any more of this candy. The mind is receiving information from the outside and dictating to the conscience. At the same time, the conscience has information that has already been programmed in. I think maybe science would call it DNA. Suddenly, we see we have a decision to make. Will I accept the information from the mind based on what is being received, or will I compare it with the information already there and then make my decision?

The unique difference between man and animal is the ability man has been given to make choices. Man has been given the responsibility to make decisions and each decision will have an impact, which will either help or hurt himself and/or creation.

That final decision will determine the success or failure of a situation. There is a saying that has passed through many circles, stated in many forms, "a house divided will fall," "united we stand, divided we fall." When we take what the mind is receiving and line it up with what is actually in the inner man or conscience, we are united. When we allow the mind to continue to process information that is not in agreement with the conscience, we cause fear and confusion. There is no question that the greatest thing to fear is fear itself.

I did not start writing to produce a book, but was simply journaling to determine what I needed to do, as well as reflect on what was happening around me during that time. When I would get discouraged, I pulled out my journal. When Trampus was "failing" at something, I would go back and read about his successes. As I meditated on the "why and why not," I would pen it so that when the answers came, I would remember that the hard times passed and light would come if I could just "wait" and "be still." That's when I would remember that "good" could and would come from every experience.

There are many things that I wish I could take care of for Trampus. Things I think he wants and that I wish I could get for him. Like, the ability to get his driver's license…I can't fix that; to have a girlfriend…I can't fix that; to run a recording and music business…I can't fix that; to grasp the concept of time, how long is a minute versus an hour versus a month? I can't fix that either. I believe we have discovered a very important truth about Trampus (possibly of others with DS as well), you can't lay a foundation and expect him to build on it like his siblings. Also we have found that he lacks the ability to make choices based on deductive reasoning.

Often times he expresses himself in reverse. By that, I mean, he may say he doesn't want to be a part of an event or activity when he really does. In fact, we decided he could be compared to the Indian in *Little Big Man*, who was contrary to the extent he rode his horse backwards. We even pursued testing for dyslexic but it proved negative.

LIFE AFTER SCHOOL

Trampus is living a wonderful life, interacting with people in our community through his job at Publix, and working with us and with our employees in the family business. He plays an important role in quality control. He is able to fold the garments properly and to verify the count of the same. He has a tremendous ability to catch errors before the product is delivered to the customer and has an unconditional loyalty to his father that no errors will slip through. We are continuously being told by those around him what a wonderful affect he has on the people that have the opportunity to be with him.

He continues to improve in his music as he practices each of his instruments. One day we get the pleasure of the trumpet, only later to enjoy the keyboard. Then come the days we hear him playing his guitar. He has a wonderful guitar instructor, John Smith, who has done a tremendous job in teaching Trampus how to play the guitar. Trampus loves John, and his love for Trampus is very evident. One of the recitals was planned at a local restaurant, Wild Wings, and Trampus was going to play "Wagon Wheel." My older son has always had an ear for music, so I suggested that he sing while Trampus played. After much persuasion, he agreed, and they were incredible. Both seem to really enjoy their ventures. We're looking forward to hearing them perform "Chicken Fried." My daughter in Florida texted me one day and asked if both boys got the music talent, "What did I get?" I was able to quickly respond with "good sense!" She just laughed.

One thing I've just recently experienced and still amazes me was the time needed for me to walk in my own learned lessons. "Never give up if it's a strong desire in your heart." Trampus has been talking about writing music for months now. He will sit down and write, and then bring it to us for approval. The real struggle is in the continuity of expressing himself. It's difficult for him to put his thoughts on paper. Our response hit hard when I realized rather than encouraging, we were trying to discourage him. We were reminding him how well he played and that writing music may not be his gift. I would see his disappointment as he walked away, with a bowed head, saying "Okay." What could I be thinking? My constant instruction is "don't give up. If you want it, keep trying." Now when he brings me his songs, I try to give a little advice, but more importantly, I try to encourage him. I am noticing he's getting better and better at it. I'm convinced now that one day he will get that song written. What an inspiration in fortitude and effort!

As I write, we are getting ready to schedule his flight to visit his sister. After he returns from Florida, it will be off to New Jersey with Special Olympics South Carolina for a National Golf Tournament. In the meantime, he works hard to save for his "apartment" that he and his father have designed. It will have a "catwalk" to our house so we will be there for him if he needs us, but he will have some independence as well. He's really excited about the "recording studio" they are designing and will be using for his world of music.

I think the most important reason I have for putting my story on paper is to take what I've learned from this child with "special needs" and cause others not only to desire to open up, but to have confidence in the ability within themselves to interact and learn from others even though they may be different. To stress the need to guard against worldly thinking that usually results in negativism, i.e., giving directions referring to the third red (stop) light rather than the third green (go) light, pointing out how many questions were missed rather than marking the ones that are correct. We can even see it when we choose to see a cup as half empty rather than half full. Again, it's helping us to see that the choices are left up to each of us individually. If we look for each one's abilities rather than deficiencies, and then work together with these abilities, we may never see a situation come up short.

The really neat thing is when we practice it in our own homes, all of our children benefit because each one has a need that may not be realized as readily as those that are more visible. There is a plan for each one of them, and certain things that we do for them and say to them may be critical in opening the doors for that plan to come to fruition. I think this is important not only in working with our own children, but when working with people in general.

Trampus has been a gift that God has provided for anyone willing to interact with him, who desires to walk in unconditional love. He is a visual tool to teach us the need for compassion, mercy, and forgiveness in each of our lives. Unfortunately, many of us have not taken the time to look within ourselves to get that reading. Trampus has also provided us the opportunity of revealing the true condition of our hearts. Thank you God for this visible gift of your love!

As I look back, I think one of the many lessons that can be learned in being with those who have special needs is the opportunity to stimulate one's own creativity, produce patience, and overall sensitivity to others. I was going through life in my own world of experiences that allowed little consideration for those who were different. My environment was protected, not necessarily by my choice, but because of society's choices; I just wasn't aware of the need to come against these choices. My greatest hope for our society is that if we can realize the importance and need we all have for each other, then we will see the need to break down barriers that require categorizing and isolation.

If you're reading my story because you have a precious little one with special needs, please do not be discouraged if you're not able to "sit in" on classes or aren't interested in music. Know most importantly that your child is special, but not just because of needs. God does not create for nothing, so the most important part you will play is to be still and listen to your "inner man." As you watch for strengths, they will become evident. Stay confident that lives around you will change as a result of your "gift," and while many will stare and back away, many more will love and embrace in a way you have never known. If you are reading it because you are teaching one, or maybe because you are a physician caring for his or her physical needs, realize the opportunities that lay before you—realize the wonderful creative side of you that can be used in this relationship. Dig down deep within yourself and use that creativity and please, most of all—savor each moment and truly enjoy the journey that is set before you. Be the encourager for that family. Be a light in what might be a dark time in their lives.

I have realized through the years that there are many roads that can be traveled to get to one destination. The same is true for the paths of our lives. I know that our road was a path found as a result of our personalities, needs, and desires. I believe the most important factor is not found based on the road taken, but rather on arriving at the desired destination.

Regardless of the route you choose to take, know without a doubt that if you embrace your desires and maintain the confidence that you have the ability to accomplish those desires, it will be a journey that will not only bring excitement, self satisfaction, and joy, but will change the lives around you as it changes you.

God bless and have a wonderful trip!